Penguin Books
The Search for the Virus

Steve Connor has a degree in zoology from the University of
Oxford. He joined *New Scientist* as deputy news editor in
1983. He is co-author of a book on surveillance, computers
and privacy entitled *On the Record* (Michael Joseph, 1986). In
1986 he won a Science Writers Fellowship.

Sharon Kingman has a degree in zoology from the University of
Durham. Since then she has worked in medical and scientific
journalism. She joined the features department of *New Scientist* in 1985, becoming science correspondent at the end of
1986.

STEVE CONNOR AND
SHARON KINGMAN

THE SEARCH
FOR THE
VIRUS

Second edition

Penguin Books

PENGUIN BOOKS

Published by the Penguin Group
27 Wrights Lane, London W8 5TZ, England
Viking Penguin Inc., 40 West 23rd Street, New York, New York 10010, USA
Penguin Books Australia Ltd, Ringwood, Victoria, Australia
Penguin Books Canada Ltd, 2801 John Street, Markham, Ontario, Canada L3R 1B4
Penguin Books (NZ) Ltd, 182–190 Wairau Road, Auckland 10, New Zealand

Penguin Books Ltd, Registered Offices: Harmondsworth, Middlesex, England

First published 1988
Second edition 1989
10 9 8 7 6 5 4 3 2 1

Filmset in Melior
Typeset, printed and bound in Great Britain by
Hazell Watson & Viney Limited
Member of BPCC plc
Aylesbury, Bucks, England

For those who died alone

CONTENTS

LIST OF FIGURES

Illustrations by Peter Gardiner

ACKNOWLEDGEMENTS

We thank the many people who have helped us to write this book. In particular, we express our gratitude to Fred Pearce, who read and made useful comments on several chapters; to Celia Dodd, who gave expert editorial advice as a non-scientist; and to Susanna Hourani and Peter Gardiner, who made helpful suggestions about parts of our early draft. We also thank the many scientists at the forefront of AIDS research who read and criticized certain chapters of the book, or took part in valuable discussions, including Michael Adler, Mike Bailey, John Barbara, Wilson Carswell, Angus Dalgleish, Anne Johnson, Myra McClure, Timothy Peto, Quentin Sattentau and Ian Weller. Fred Brown and Don Jeffries gave valuable advice for the second edition. All opinions and errors, of course, remain our own. Caroline Akehurst, David Fitzsimons and Renée Sabatier provided useful assistance. Special thanks are also due to Amanda Robinson, for her practical help. Omar Sattaur carried out much of the early groundwork on the subject. Christopher Joyce and Ian Anderson provided important research material from the United States. Michael Kenward encouraged us to start the project in the first place, as well as commenting on our manuscript. Finally, we thank our colleagues on *New Scientist* who have tolerated our preoccupation with AIDS.

Chapter 1

AN INFECTION OF IGNORANCE

We could not have designed a more frightening disease if we had tried. If we could play at being Satan for the day, charged with the task of designing an epidemic to undermine both the developed and underdeveloped countries of the world at the end of the twentieth century, then the blueprint for the design would incorporate many of the features of AIDS. An artificial pestilence would have to have all the subtleties and idiosyncrasies of acquired immune deficiency syndrome – AIDS – in order to kill the maximum number of people and cause untold disruption to the health services of countries throughout the world.

A modern plague has a greater chance of spreading if it can be transmitted during the most intimate and compulsive of human activities – sex. Science can fight disease with the cooperation of those at risk of infection, but a disease that spreads with the help of sex is a formidable foe. There are few occasions in history when laws have successfully stopped people from having sexual relations with each other. And in modern society, sex has gone international. People travel more now than ever before, and sexual relationships have crossed national boundaries. Sex has even become a tourist attraction. Yet, despite the sexual liberation that has marked the latter half of the twentieth century, sex is still a surreptitious activity, so the hypothetical designers of a modern

1

plague can take advantage of the age-old taboos that are still associated with sex. The shame of sex and the reluctance even to admit its existence is, after all, as ancient as the story of forbidden fruit in the Garden of Eden.

A modern plague would have to be more subtle and complex than previous diseases in order to outwit modern medical science. It would have to attack an important and yet vulnerable part of the body. AIDS does this. The virus that causes AIDS attacks and destroys the immune system, which is responsible for fighting off infections. Without the immune system, the human body cannot fend off even the most trivial illnesses, and it becomes an open target for hundreds of potentially deadly organisms. AIDS results from the inability of the body to defend itself from infection. A person without an effective immune system becomes easy prey to a myriad of microorganisms.

The structure of the AIDS virus is almost perfect. For a start, in common with all viruses, it is tiny; so small that its simple structure cannot be said to be living because it can only replicate by hijacking a living cell. A virus therefore straddles the divide between living and non-living matter. The virus lives and replicates within human cells, a perfect place to escape from the body's defences. Most viruses do this, which is why they are so effective. The virus that causes AIDS, however, performs an even neater trick: it becomes part of the genetic material of the cell. Hiding within this innermost sanctum of our bodies, the virus adopts the ultimate camouflage – it becomes part of the person it infects.

Cloistered away like this, the virus becomes quiescent. Its dormancy can last months or even years. People who carry the virus during this time have few, if any, obvious symptoms of infection. Some may never go on to develop the hotchpotch collection of diseases, such as skin cancer, pneumonia, and other infections, that comprise acquired immune deficiency syndrome. (These terminal infections signal 'full-blown' AIDS.) People without the early signs of AIDS can nevertheless still pass the virus to others. With no symptoms to alert them, carriers can be completely unaware that they

2

are spawning further generations of viruses. A designer of a modern plague would admire this characteristic of AIDS, too. The long delay between the moment of infection and the appearance of the symptoms of AIDS secures the stealthy spread of the virus throughout the population.

Another strength of the virus is its ability to change its structure with each generation. The body's immune system relies heavily on being able to recognize microorganisms from their outer coatings. The AIDS virus mutates very fast, so fast that it becomes exceedingly difficult to identify any similarities between the outer coat of one individual virus and the coat of another. The result is that the body cannot launch a successful attack against this constantly moving target. This detail completes the frustratingly perfect design of the virus that causes AIDS.

The perfection, however, does not end with the virus, nor with how it spreads from person to person. Other aspects of AIDS make it difficult for modern science to tackle. There are further prejudices and taboos, not just about sex, but about sexual preferences, lifestyles, drug addiction, race and nationality. These prejudices combine to make AIDS the ultimate vehicle for transporting fear, hysteria, hatred and panic around the four corners of the globe. If scientists could not have designed a better disease, then psychologists could not have designed a better mechanism for provoking irrational reactions and disturbing the human psyche.

The story of AIDS is full of examples of ignorance. This ignorance has led to confusion and fear, which in turn have developed into distrust and hatred. AIDS does not spread by casual contact. People cannot become infected with the virus by handling the clothing of people with the disease or by shaking hands with them. AIDS is not, in short, a highly contagious disease, so it is not strictly speaking a 'modern plague', equivalent to the Black Death which decimated Europe in the Middle Ages.

Medical scientists became concerned about the early press reports on AIDS, which often described the disease as the

3

'gay plague'. The press coverage seemed to be encouraging irrational fears: people were being led to believe that they could catch AIDS by merely associating with sufferers. As a dozen of the world's leading figures in medical virology and infectious diseases made clear at a meeting at the World Health Organization in Geneva in September 1985, one of the greatest threats of AIDS arises from ignorance, in particular ignorance about how the disease spreads. The chairman of the meeting, Professor Friedrich Deinhardt, a leading virologist from the Max von Pettenkofer Institute in Munich, said at the time: 'In no way can AIDS be compared to the great plague of the Middle Ages. There is no evidence that it is spread through casual contact with an infected person. It is primarily a sexually transmitted disease.'

Scientists wanted to nip the growing hysteria about AIDS in the bud. It would take a long time for the message to seep in. Part of the problem was that far too many people in a position to know better were still confused about how AIDS can spread from one person to another.

Such ignorance fuelled the existing prejudice against homosexuals and other groups associated with AIDS. Examples of the hysteria range from the serious to the trivial. In 1985, telephone engineers initially refused to mend the equipment at Gay Switchboard in London. The engineers said that they might catch AIDS from the telephones. More seriously, AIDS has become the pretext for a combination of assaults on gay men. On the streets, homosexuals have been attacked and abused, and in government, politicians have devised a number of draconian measures designed to 'curb AIDS' by discriminating against gay men and women.

Haemophiliacs, who suffer from a clotting disorder of the blood for which they need treatment which may put them at risk of AIDS, did not escape such discrimination. Haemophiliac children were ostracized by their schoolfriends. Worse still, some parents of healthy children tried to stop haemophiliacs from attending the same school as their children. In Indiana in the US, for instance, pressure from parents prevented a nine-year-old haemophiliac boy from attending

4

lessons. In a similar case in New York, parents kept thousands of children at home as a protest at the local school authorities permitting children with AIDS to attend classes. In Britain, and other European countries, similar concern grew about the perceived danger that haemophiliacs posed to other children. In one school in Hampshire in southern England, for instance, many parents kept their children at home for fear of their catching AIDS from a pupil at the school, a small boy with haemophilia.

The British government came under pressure from the worried parents of haemophiliac children. The Department of Health issued a pamphlet to teachers in March 1986 explaining that children with the AIDS virus should be treated no differently from other children, and could take part in school activities in the usual way. This leaflet explained that there is a danger of children passing on the virus in blood, so teachers should discourage any behaviour that may result in bleeding, such as tattooing, ear piercing or 'blood-brother' rituals. In many cases, however, the advice did little to quell the growing fear of other children and their parents.

The fear of AIDS has resulted in hysterical reactions in supposedly well-educated and well-informed groups of people. For example, the university dons at one Oxford college banned a centuries-old tradition of passing a 'loving cup' of wine around the table at the college's annual dinner. They thought the ban would be prudent given that 'certain diseases' were rife, even though there was no scientific evidence that the virus could spread in saliva. In the US, the National Science Foundation announced in 1987 that scientists wanting to spend the winter at its research post in the Antarctic must have a blood test for infection with the AIDS virus. The regulation did not apply to scientists wanting to spend summer there — it appears that even some scientifically trained people were under the impression that sex only takes place after dark.

Police officers have also overreacted to AIDS. In 1988, police in Scotland burned and then compressed a car that had been stolen by a person thought to be infected with the virus, on the grounds that the thief was involved in an accident and had bled profusely. In another incident involving a thief, a householder burned his bed and bedclothes after an intruder had taken a nap during a burglary at the house.

Accusations of overreaction have been levelled at medical authorities. For example, in 1987 some Scottish medical schools advised students not to go to African countries for fear of infection with the AIDS virus. Several doctors from the same medical schools pointed out in letters to the British medical journal, the *Lancet*, that the risk of acquiring AIDS as a result of emergency treatment with unsterilized surgical instruments or contaminated blood is more remote than the usual risks associated with travelling in tropical climates. Two of these doctors, Arnold Klopper and Nicholas Fisk of the University of Aberdeen, wrote: 'It is a remarkable coincidence that such controversial advice should have been issued simultaneously by three or four Scottish medical schools . . . To ask us to ostracize our colleagues in Africa is a serious matter. It marks a profound departure in university attitudes and policy.'

African countries have borne the brunt of a rising tide of xenophobia resulting from the spread of AIDS. Many governments outside Africa have stipulated that foreigners must have a test for infection with the AIDS virus before they can enter and stay in the country in question. Very often the testing regimes were ill-disguised attempts to take unnecessary and arbitrary action against visitors and students from African countries. India, for example, initially wanted to test African students resident in the country. The Indian government later amended this to all new students, because of the blatantly discriminatory nature of the initial plan.

Throughout the world, governments have moved to stem the spread of AIDS. A common thread running through the laws that they have enacted is the belief that testing foreigners will somehow limit the incidence of AIDS at home. In Britain the government resisted a vociferous campaign to test black immigrants. The campaign reached a shrill climax with the leaking of a 'Whitehall report' to the *Sunday Telegraph* in

September 1986. The report was evidently a collection of impressions of British diplomats stationed in several countries in Central Africa. The author of the report, which went to the Foreign Secretary, suggested that visitors from Africa 'could be a primary source of infection and should be subject to compulsory tests'. An editorial in the *Sunday Telegraph* articulated the paper's position:

'It would be monstrous if ministers were to hold back from action lest they be accused of racial discrimination. For in this instance, there is a positive duty to discriminate. In the matter of AIDS, black Africa does have a uniquely bad record and only harm can spring from pretending otherwise.' (The editorial invoked the familiar theme of invading black hordes. It said: 'In a few days' time, hundreds of students from Zambia, Uganda and Tanzania will be arriving in this country. A significant proportion of them – possibly up to 10 per cent – could be AIDS carriers.')

The real pretence, however, was that countries could somehow close the stable doors after the horse had bolted. Britain by this time already had a significant number of people infected with the virus, and most of them had had no contact whatsoever with 'black Africa'.

In the US, the country with more documented cases of AIDS than any other, the same irrational view came to the fore in May 1987 with the first speech on AIDS by President Ronald Reagan. Before a glittering dinner held at the Potomac Hotel in Washington DC to raise funds for the American Foundation for AIDS Research, chaired by the actress Elizabeth Taylor, Reagan upset many scientists by saying that he supported routine testing for infection with the AIDS virus as part of a programme for discriminating against those found to be infected. The medical establishment had already concluded that routine testing was impractical, expensive and next to useless. Yet Reagan said:

'I have asked the Department of Health and Human Services (HHS) to determine as soon as possible the extent to which the AIDS virus has penetrated our society and to predict its future dimensions. I have also asked HHS to add the AIDS virus to the list of contagious diseases for which immigrants and aliens seeking permanent residence in the United States can be denied entry.' By the following month, June 1987, the US had classified AIDS as a dangerous 'contagious' disease under the Immigration and Nationality Act. Anyone suffering from AIDS would be denied permanent entry into the US. Furthermore, the US government also decided to consider classifying people infected with the virus, but without AIDS, in the same category. Many scientists, however, were still not convinced of the usefulness of blood tests as a technique for mass testing. A negative test, for instance, is not proof that the person is not infected. And when screening a large group of people for a virus that is very rare, there is a strong chance of wrongly identifying uninfected people as 'positive'.

Countries with diverse political complexions have taken very similar stands on testing foreign visitors. South Africa, for example, announced in 1987 that all immigrants, including hundreds of thousands of black migrant workers, would have to have tests. Those found positive would be expelled. Any citizen can be tested, and quarantining is permitted. Cuba has drawn up similar plans to test foreign visitors. In addition, the Cuban Deputy Minister of Health, Hector Terry, said in 1987 that all of Cuba's ten million citizens will be tested by 1989. Terry has issued warnings to Cubans to 'avoid fortuitous contacts with foreigners', whatever that may mean. Meanwhile, the country has already begun to quarantine its own citizens who have AIDS.

In China, fear of AIDS and of foreigners resulted in a government campaign to burn imported second-hand clothes. In November 1985, a crowd of city officials from Beijing, including the city's deputy mayor, watched a group of soldiers with flamethrowers incinerate twenty tonnes of second-hand clothes imported from Japan, Hong Kong and Macao. The officials feared that the clothes harboured the AIDS virus.

In the Soviet Union, the Presidium of the Supreme Soviet, the highest authority in the country, took the necessary legislative steps to ensure that rigorous measures could be taken against anyone, foreign or native, infected with the AIDS virus. The Presidium adopted a decree in August 1987 stating:

The citizens of the USSR, as well as foreign citizens and stateless persons living or staying in the territory of the USSR, may be bound to take a medical test for the AIDS virus. If they dodge the test voluntarily, the persons, in relation of whom there are grounds for assuming that they are infected with the AIDS virus, may be brought to medical institutions by health authorities with the assistance, in the necessary cases, of authorities from the interior ministry.

The decree stated that anyone infected with the virus who is found to have deliberately exposed other people to the virus would be imprisoned for up to five years. For knowingly giving AIDS to someone else, the maximum prison sentence is eight years.

Soon after the government issued this decree, the Soviet authorities put the new law into action. In September 1987, more than a hundred foreign visitors were expelled from the country. All but three were from Central Africa. In the same month, a twenty-eight-year-old Soviet woman had to make a pledge to refrain from sexual relations for an arbitrary period of five years because she was diagnosed as being infected with the AIDS virus. If she broke the pledge, her punishment would be a prison sentence of up to eight years. All Soviet citizens returning from a foreign visit lasting more than four weeks have to have a blood test for infection. This even applies to Soviet AIDS researchers who collaborate with foreign scientists.

Many countries in the West have also discussed what to do about people who are infected with the virus and who knowingly put others at risk. In West Germany, courts in the state of Bavaria jailed a prostitute in 1987 for continuing her trade when she knew she had the AIDS virus. In the same state, an American civilian was accused of grievous bodily harm for having sexual intercourse even though he knew that he was infected. In November 1987, the courts sent the man to prison for two years. In Switzerland, doctors are obliged by law to tell health authorities about all cases of infection, not just cases of AIDS. The rule, which became law in 1987, marked a new departure for countries in Western Europe, some of which had shied away from making it obligatory to notify even cases of AIDS because of worries about the confidentiality of the information.

Ever since the problem of AIDS first arose, Britain has tussled with the issue of whether to make AIDS a 'notifiable' disease. This would make it compulsory for doctors to notify local authorities of patients with AIDS, and could also give hospitals the right to apply for a court order to detain patients against their will if necessary. In early 1985, the government considered making AIDS notifiable but, after taking advice from his committee of experts, the Minister of Health at the time, Kenneth Clarke, did not think this was necessary. However, Clarke said in February 1985:

There might be very rare and exceptional cases where the nature of a patient's condition would place him in a dangerously infectious state which would make it desirable to admit him to, or detain him in, hospital . . . It is my intention therefore to lay regulations under the Public Health (Control of Disease) Act 1984 which would give reserve powers to authorities to detain a patient when he is in a dangerously infectious condition . . . We need these reserve powers for the very rare case that might eventually arise somewhere sometime.

Such a case arose seven months later, in September 1985. A twenty-nine-year-old man suffering from AIDS in a Manchester hospital became the first person in Britain to be detained against his will because he had AIDS. The hospital authorities had applied for a court order because the patient was 'bleeding copiously and trying to discharge himself' from hospital. The court order had the backing of Britain's chief medical officer, Donald Acheson, who felt that 'in the circumstances it would be too risky for [the patient] to leave the hospital'. The court eventually lifted the order after an appeal and a promise by the patient to stay in hospital and to continue treatment.

In the US, a vociferous campaign to incarcerate AIDS sufferers gathered momentum after doctors found that the disease had begun to spread to groups outside the gay community. At least one American senator was heard to say that 'somewhere along the line we are going to have to quarantine'. In November 1986, Californians voted on a new law, dubbed 'Proposition 64', that would, if enacted, make it compulsory for doctors to report people carrying the virus or suffering from the disease. The supporters of the proposition, the Prevent AIDS Now Initiative Committee (who did not worry about being called by their acronym, PANIC) wanted no carrier of the virus to be a teacher, employee or student of a university or school in the state. They also called on authorities to 'quarantine [people] as much as required to stop the spread of the disease'. Compulsory reporting would be necessary in order to identify the people to lock up.

A powerful supporter of Proposition 64 was Lyndon LaRouche, a right-wing political figure in the United States. He justified the proposal with a number of 'facts'. Medical research, LaRouche said, had proved that biting insects spread AIDS, and that people can pass on AIDS by 'casual contact'. Medical research had proved nothing of the sort, and when Californians voted on Proposition 64 on 4 November 1986, they threw it out. This came as a ray of hope for those who feared that ignorance was beginning to dominate the battle against AIDS. After all, only five years earlier, science had been on the brink of overcoming one of the main obstacles to fighting AIDS – ignorance of its existence.

Chapter 2

DIAGNOSIS OF A DISEASE

The title of the first scientific paper on AIDS gave little away: 'Pneumocystis pneumonia – Los Angeles'. The article was published on 5 June 1981, in a then relatively obscure American journal called *Morbidity and Mortality Weekly Report* (*MMWR*). It did not mention the word AIDS. Within a year of that article being published, doctors in the US began to realize that an epidemic of mysterious illnesses had appeared in young, mainly homosexual, men.

Michael Gottlieb and Wayne Shandera knew that something strange was happening to some of their patients. Gottlieb, a doctor with the University of California at Los Angeles, had come across four cases of an exceedingly rare type of pneumonia, which was caused by an infection with a microorganism called *Pneumocystis carinii* in the lungs. All four patients were young men in their late twenties or early thirties, and all were homosexual. Gottlieb spoke to his colleague Shandera, of the Los Angeles County Department of Public Health, about the unusual outbreak. Shandera looked at his own records and found that his department had a similar case. This patient was homosexual as well. So there were five cases of *Pneumocystis* pneumonia in the same area, at the same time, and in a group of men who were all young homosexuals. Gottlieb and Shandera wondered if they had discovered a new epidemic.

Realizing the sensitivity of discovering a potential 'gay disease', the *MMWR* published a vapid account of their work. 'The patients did not know each other and had no known common contacts or knowledge of sexual partners who had had similar illnesses.' An editorial note at the end of this short report said that the occurrence of *Pneumocystis* pneumonia in the US was almost exclusively limited to patients who had undergone some sort of therapy which had, as a side effect, severely depleted the number of their white blood cells – an important component of their immune systems. The result is immune suppression, also known as immunodeficiency. A suppressed immune system is seriously weakened to such an extent that infections can take hold of the body. The editorial note continued: 'The occurrence of pneumocystosis in these five previously healthy individuals without a clinically apparent underlying immunodeficiency is unusual.'

A month later, on 4 July 1981, another report appeared in the *MMWR*, which is the journal of the organization responsible for monitoring the health of Americans, the Centers for Disease Control, in Atlanta, Georgia. The CDC had gathered together a number of intriguing reports from doctors on both the west and east coasts of America. These doctors had found a very rare type of skin cancer, called Kaposi's sarcoma, in twenty-six homosexual men: twenty from New York City and six from California.

What made the Centers for Disease Control interested in these reports was the age of the men concerned. They were all much younger than the patients who normally developed Kaposi's sarcoma. (This type of skin cancer usually affects men in their seventies, and then tends to develop only in men of certain racial groups, mainly of Mediterranean ancestry.) Seven of the patients had infections as well as the skin cancer – four had *Pneumocystis* pneumonia, just like the five homosexual men that Gottlieb had reported a month earlier. Furthermore, since the publication of Gottlieb's account, doctors in California had found an additional ten cases of *Pneumocystis* pneumonia in homosexual men.

An editorial in the *Morbidity and Mortality Weekly Report*

13

pointed to the extraordinary nature of the observations: 'The occurrence of this number of Kaposi's sarcoma cases during a thirty-month period among young homosexual men is considered highly unusual. No previous association between Kaposi's sarcoma and sexual preference has been reported.'

The CDC decided to set up a task-force to investigate these strange illnesses. One avenue of inquiry was to search through the CDC's files for cases where doctors had prescribed a drug called pentamidine. This drug is often effective against *Pneumocystis* pneumonia. Past prescriptions for pentamidine, which the CDC collates centrally for the whole of the US, revealed the existence of more cases of this form of pneumonia among young men. But few cases had occurred before 1979, indicating that the 'epidemic' was a very recent one.

Further work by the CDC, published in August 1981 in the *MMWR*, confirmed a link between *Pneumocystis* pneumonia and Kaposi's sarcoma: 'The apparent clustering of both *Pneumocystis carinii* pneumonia and Kaposi's sarcoma among homosexual men suggests a common underlying factor.' A year later, in 1982, the CDC came to the conclusion that something was affecting the immune systems of these patients, so permitting 'opportunistic infections'. These are infections which the body can normally shrug off but which take advantage of a weak immune system. An early name for the condition was gay related immune deficiency syndrome – GRIDS. Later, in 1982, the CDC changed this to acquired immune deficiency syndrome, or AIDS, because people other than homosexual men also began to develop the condition. The doctors thought 'AIDS' suitable because people acquired the condition rather than inherited it, because it results in a deficiency within the immune system, and because it is a syndrome, with a number of manifestations, rather than a single disease.

Throughout 1982, and subsequent years, the researchers at the CDC continued to collect details on more and more cases of AIDS. The syndrome began to affect women as well as men, haemophiliacs as well as homosexuals, and children as well as adults. A crisis was unfolding.

The World Health Organization estimated that the virus responsible for causing AIDS had by 1987 infected between five million and ten million people. By late 1988, the WHO had received reports of more than 124,000 cases of AIDS in 142 countries. This figure, the organization said, represents 'only a fraction of the total cases' of AIDS. In 1988, the WHO estimated that the true figure for the total number of cases of AIDS to date was in the region of 200,000 to 250,000. The reason for the discrepancy is that some countries have difficulties in reporting and diagnosing people suffering from the various illnesses that make up acquired immune deficiency syndrome.

The 'hidden pandemic' of AIDS has forced the WHO to establish a special programme to tackle the disease, especially in developing countries of the Third World. The organization believes that by 1991, one million people on the globe will suffer from AIDS, placing an extraordinary burden on the health services of the developed world, and possibly bringing about the economic collapse of certain countries in the Third World. The director of the WHO's programme on AIDS, Jonathan Mann, spoke about the problem at a scientific conference in Washington DC in 1987. He said that an analysis of the numbers of people estimated to be infected with the AIDS virus and a look at the numbers of people suffering from the symptoms of AIDS led him to the 'virtually inescapable conclusion that we are imminently facing a precipitous increase in the number of AIDS cases'. He continued: 'If five to ten million persons are currently infected [with the AIDS virus] worldwide, and assuming that 10–30 per cent of these persons will develop AIDS during the next five years, then from 500,000 to three million new AIDS cases will emerge from persons already infected with [the virus]. Compared with the number of AIDS cases reported thus far, a more than ten-fold increase in AIDS cases may be anticipated during the next five years.' That was in 1987.

In his speech, Mann referred to the 'two epidemics' of AIDS – the first being the realization that the virus has infected a large proportion of a given population, and the second being the inevitable consequence of this: people start dying of AIDS. The 'third epidemic', he said, follows the first two. 'This is the epidemic of economic, social and political and cultural reaction and response to . . . AIDS.' AIDS is in many ways different to many of the epidemics that the WHO has had to deal with. Most public-health problems in the past have affected either the very young or the very old. But AIDS affects, as Mann said, 'the most vital segment of the population in terms of social and economic development. The selective involvement of young and middle-aged adults, including business and government cadres and members of social, economic and political élites, leads to potential for economic and political destabilization'. What political system, Mann asked in 1987, could withstand up to 25 per cent of its young adults dying of AIDS?

The United States is the richest nation on Earth yet the figures suggest that even the US will find it increasingly difficult to meet the economic as well as the social costs of AIDS. By the end of 1987, the CDC estimated that up to 1·5 million Americans could be infected with the virus. At that time almost 50,000 Americans had developed AIDS, and many of them had already died. One year later, the figure had risen above 70,000. The US Institute of Medicine predicts that by 1991 this figure will have leapt to 270,000, with 179,000 deaths. The institute believes that in 1991 alone doctors will diagnose 74,000 new cases of AIDS – equivalent to the population of a small town. In the same year, the institute predicts, over 50,000 Americans will die of AIDS. By this stage, most people will personally know of someone who has developed the disease.

There will be regions in the US where the situation will be much worse. Some cities have already reached a crisis. Since 1984, for example, AIDS has become the biggest single cause of death among men aged between thirty and thirty-nine living in New York City. By 1987, AIDS had also become the

16

number-one killer among women aged between twenty-five and thirty-four in the same city. Other cities in the US and elsewhere in the world will inevitably follow the trend. An editorial in the *Journal of the American Medical Association*, in September 1987, described the prospects for the US:

'The loss of human life is staggering. By 1991, AIDS will be among the top ten leading causes of death in the United States, far exceeding all other causes of death for people between the ages of twenty-five and forty-four years. Socially, politically and economically, AIDS is an ever-worsening disaster.'

In 1981, the year that scientists first discovered a condition they later called 'AIDS', the US government spent $200,000 on the disease. The government was pressed to increase this allocation to $1·145 billion by 1989, two thirds to be spent on medical research to find a vaccine and a cure, and the other third designated for prevention and health education.

The costs to the US, however, of an ever-rising number of people falling ill with AIDS and needing medical treatment are truly staggering. Accountants in the US government estimated in 1987 that the total cost of medical treatment for AIDS sufferers will reach $8,500m in 1991, which will be 1.4 per cent of the nation's total health bill. In 1985, AIDS soaked up just 0.2 per cent of this national expenditure. The same accountants, from the US General Accounting Office, came up with a more worrying calculation. They estimated the amount of money the American economy will lose as a result of young working people dying prematurely of AIDS and calculated that this sum will come to more than $55,000m by 1991. Even this staggering figure is an underestimate, as accountants did not include days lost from work due to the variety of illnesses people contract before they develop full-blown AIDS. The accountants also based their calculation on the assumption that just 20–30 per cent of the people infected with the virus will go on to develop AIDS, which many scientists believe is a conservative figure. They believe it could be far higher.

A study by American researchers in September 1987 found

that it cost annually $20,000 on average to look after an AIDS patient who had to spend short periods each year in an American hospital. The researchers came to this conclusion after surveying about 5,400 hospital patients with AIDS two years previously. The researchers, who published their findings in the *Journal of the American Medical Association*, concluded: 'Our results portend possible catastrophic effects on both government and private payers as health-care costs of AIDS escalate.' The journal said in an editorial in the same issue: 'The tremendous costs of this particular disease are exacerbating the problems of an already flawed health-care system . . . Who, then, is going to pay the costs?' Other researchers, basing their estimates of health-care costs on 270,000 cases diagnosed between 1981 and 1991, said that the US would have a $22m health bill by 1991 due to AIDS. Some American cities will find the economic burden unbearable. Some individuals will find health insurance difficult or impossible to obtain, putting great stress on the US's Medicaid system of public insurance.

Even the enormous sums that the US government had earmarked in 1987 for AIDS were not going to be enough, according to the report on the disease by the accountants from the General Accounting Office. The spending plans of the US government for projects to prevent the spread of AIDS, in particular, were 'not adequate'. Many specialists involved in fighting AIDS thought that 'perceived lack of federal leadership' was making matters worse and was 'at least as troublesome as estimated shortfalls in the budget'. The US Institute of Medicine had told the General Accounting Office that many students showed an 'alarming degree of misinformation' about AIDS. 'As late as 1986,' the GAO's report stated, 'even students in San Francisco were seriously misinformed about routes of transmission and preventive practices. Specifically, 40 per cent did not know that AIDS is caused by a virus or that the use of a condom during sexual intercourse decreases the risk of transmitting [the virus].'

The US government has shown a startling degree of indifference to the epidemic, even though AIDS had, according to official figures, claimed more lives in America than the rest of the world put together. It took six years for President Reagan to make a pronouncement on the disease, and a presidential commission he set up in July 1987 was immediately criticized for being preoccupied with morals rather than with tactics to fight AIDS. Many people believed the commission did not fully represent the high-risk groups, notably gays, most in need of a voice in government. Neither did it have enough scientific expertise. The chairman of the commission was forced to resign just two months after taking office after disagreements emerged within the commission itself. Many scientists and others working on AIDS thought that the commission lacked both expertise and objectivity.

Eventually the commission reported to Reagan in June 1988. The new chairman, retired admiral James D. Watkins, said that the President 'should immediately declare the [AIDS] epidemic a public health emergency' and that the Surgeon General, America's top health official, should devote all his time and energy to directing this response. Watkins said that the American government had 'thwarted' a 'timely response' to the AIDS epidemic in the US. 'Quick decisions based on newly discovered facts about the epidemic have been virtually impossible,' he said. The President's reaction to the commission's report was lukewarm. The report's recommendations fell victim to a lameduck administration waiting for a general election.

Earlier, in October 1987, the US government was due to have sent a leaflet on AIDS through the mail to every American household, which most countries in Europe had already done. The brochure, called 'America Responds to AIDS', failed to go out at the allotted time because of disagreements within the administration on how best to educate the American public about the disease. The presidential commission agreed to postpone the plan. Its former chairman, W. Eugene Mayberry, told the American journal *Science*, 'we just felt like we weren't ready to tackle the mailing yet'. In comparison to leaflets produced by other governments, notably in Europe, 'America Responds to AIDS' was hardly an explicit piece of literature. As *Science* said, 'the word "homosexual" does not put in an appearance, even though homosexuals comprise 70 per cent of AIDS cases'. Words such as 'family' appeared more frequently than words such as 'condom'.

Eventually, in the summer of 1988, a leaflet called 'Understanding AIDS' did go to every one of the US's 107 million households. The leaflet was hailed as a good explanation of the risks from AIDS. It was only a pity, some scientists remarked, that it came several years too late for thousands of Americans.

The failure of the Reagan administration to coordinate a nationwide education campaign early in the AIDS epidemic stands in stark contrast to the dire warnings issued by the administration's senior advisers. The Surgeon-General of the US, C. Everett Koop, said after the World Health Assembly in Geneva in May 1987: 'There's no doubt about the fact that most of us here who are in public health believe that we are facing the greatest challenge perhaps that public health ever faced.' Even the US Secretary of Health in 1987, Otis Bowen, had to agree. AIDS, he said, 'could well become one of the worst health problems in the history of the world . . . an awesome health problem that could involve millions of people who are going to die as a result'. The US government as a whole, however, seemed strangely oblivious to this prophecy.

Elsewhere in the developed world, the scourge of AIDS had not, by 1987, become anything like as severe as in America. Nevertheless, when doctors looked hard, they discovered that an epidemic was quietly developing. France, which then had more documented cases of AIDS than any other country apart from the US, reported its two thousandth case by the middle of 1987. But by the end of that year, Brazil was vying with France for runner-up position to the US in the AIDS league table. The silent epidemic had emerged as a strong threat in South America.

In Britain, health authorities reported the thousandth case of the disease towards the end of 1987. By the end of 1988, the tally had doubled. The problem of AIDS in the US still dwarfed that in Britain. Nevertheless, the British government had no cause to cheer. Health economists in Whitehall forecast dire consequences for the National Health Service if the numbers of people suffering from AIDS followed the American trend. Officials within the Department of Health had initially warned the government that the cost of treating someone with AIDS would be about £10,000 a year. This was bad enough. A later analysis of the real costs found that this figure was a serious underestimate. The government heard that the true cost of treating an AIDS patient was more like £20,000 a year and this would increase to over £25,000 a year if new, expensive drugs became available for therapy. The government's advisers were forecasting that the cost of treatment could accelerate almost as swiftly as the numbers that would need therapy.

The threat of hundreds of people dying and of the financial burden this would place on the health service, forced the government to set up a special Cabinet committee in 1986. Lord Whitelaw chaired the committee, which was to coordinate the government's response to the disease. The committee included ministers and advisers from most of the departments of government – Health, Foreign Office, Home Office, Education and Science, Defence and, perhaps the most important department of all, the Treasury. Scientists from the Medical Research Council met the committee regularly to keep Whitelaw and other ministers up to date on scientific developments. The Cabinet committee set several precedents. It was the first to be established to tackle a specific disease, and the first to operate in the glare of publicity (the British government normally keeps even the existence of Cabinet committees a secret).

One of the most worrying aspects about AIDS, which the committee soon realized, was the uncertainty of the predictions made by the government's scientific advisers about the course of the epidemic in Britain. An early attempt to gauge the extent of the AIDS problem, made in 1985 by researchers from the Communicable Disease Surveillance Centre

(Britain's equivalent to the Centers for Disease Control in the US), which monitors infectious diseases, predicted that 1,800 people would develop AIDS in 1988. The trouble with this informed guess, however, was that the scientists admitted that they could have got it dramatically wrong. There was a one in twenty chance, they said, that the actual number of new cases in 1988 would be less than 460 or greater than 7,300. To the politician having to make decisions concerning resources for the next few years these margins of error are very worrisome indeed. In fact, the actual number of new cases of AIDS in 1988 for Britain turned out to be about 1,000. At the end of 1988, government advisers said that up to 50,000 Britons could be infected with the virus. They told the government to expect up to 30,000 cases of AIDS by 1992 – a fifteen-fold increase in just five years.

Whitelaw and his colleagues wanted to know about the extra financial burden that AIDS would put on the state in the years to come. One organization had already assessed the problem. The Office of Health Economics, a private body funded by the drug industry, had estimated, in 1986, that Britain would spend between £20m and £30m on treating AIDS patients by 1988. 'But these figures might substantially misrepresent the eventual cost,' the office said unhelpfully. Medical journals had by then already warned that if the government did not treat the growing epidemic of AIDS seriously, then the numbers of people dying from the disease could equal the deaths resulting from the crash of a fully laden jumbo jet each month. The Office of Health Economics suggested another comparison if the government continued its 'crisis-management approach'. The office warned: 'Retrospective judgement might then suggest that an annual loss of life equivalent to four Titanic disasters would have been a more appropriate analogy.'

One of Britain's first responses to the impending threat posed by AIDS was to establish in February 1985 an advisory group of scientists, doctors and health officials. One of the group's first decisions was to tell the government that there was no need at that time to make the disease notifiable. The group's other roles included advising government about guidelines for medical staff dealing with AIDS patients, and promoting health education for the general public and those at risk of AIDS. It also advised on the screening of blood for the AIDS virus and ways of dealing with the problem of contamination of factor VIII, the clotting agent needed by haemophiliacs.

The advisory group warned the government that it needed to spend more money on fighting AIDS. By September 1985, the Department of Health realized that AIDS was beginning to burn a large hole in the coffers of health authorities in London, which had the heaviest load of AIDS patients. The department allocated an extra £1m, mainly for London, and promised to investigate the possibility of launching a national campaign to educate the public about AIDS.

At the end of 1985 the Secretary of State for Social Services, Norman Fowler, announced that he was preparing a 'package' of measures to tackle AIDS, including an information campaign costing £2.5m. The money would pay for a campaign that was to begin in the spring of 1986 and run throughout that year. Fowler said: 'The campaign will be directed at the public in general and this will be coupled with a series of targeted campaigns for those known to be at special risk. The aim is to improve understanding of the disease and the ways in which its spread can be controlled.'

Scientists were still not convinced, however, that the government was really doing all that it could at this time. Professor Julian Peto, an epidemiologist at the Institute of Cancer Research in London, told the *Observer*: 'The country is just sitting back waiting for half a million people to be infected, instead of the 10,000 or so that we have at present . . . We are heading inexorably towards an AIDS crisis like the one in America today.' At that time, at the end of 1986, the government had just introduced screening of blood donations, and many organizations were concerned that the government was not spending enough money on adequate counselling of people who proved positive for infection with the virus. David Miller, a psychologist and counsellor for the

23

hospital that then had more AIDS patients than any other in Britain, St Mary's in London, said: 'Like everyone else trying to deal with AIDS, we are having to compete fiercely for funds. It is a real uphill battle . . . The longer it takes to get that money, the further behind we get and the more unnecessary cases of AIDS develop as a result.' Jonathan Weber, another scientist from the same hospital, summed up the feelings of many professionals having to cope with the growing problem of AIDS at that time: 'Despite repeated warnings, the government has shown no intention of planning for the future.'

By the time the General Election had arrived, in the spring of 1987, the British government had become wise to this persistent criticism. It had already instigated a national advertising campaign, with commercials on television and the press warning people not to 'die of ignorance'. And just before the election, and a day before a by-election, the government announced that it was giving £14.5m to the Medical Research Council specifically for a 'directed programme' of scientific research into AIDS. It was a welcome sweetener for the council, which could not remember the last time that the British government had given medical research all that it had asked for. In less than three years, the government's attitude to funding research into AIDS had changed. Asked at the end of 1984 whether the government would allocate additional funds for research into AIDS through the Medical Research Council, Peter Brooke, a junior minister, had replied: 'It is for the Medical Research Council to decide on its scientific priorities within the resources available to it.' At that time, the council had less than £500,000 to spend on AIDS research. By late 1988, the council was expecting to spend £14m on its programme of research during 1991–92. Science in Britain had finally received the tonic it needed to enter the battle against AIDS. In France and America, scientists had already been working for quite some time on one of the most intriguing mysteries of AIDS. They were already searching for the virus.

Chapter 3

RACE FOR DISCOVERY

When scientists first discovered AIDS, they knew nothing of what was really behind the handful of diseases that eventually killed the sufferers. Initially, all they knew was that the people with AIDS fell into recognizable 'risk groups', such as homosexuals or drug users who injected their addiction. All these patients had one thing in common – their immune systems, the body's mechanism for fighting off infections, had all but collapsed. One particular white blood cell, called the T-helper cell, or 'T-cell', is an important part of the immune system. In AIDS patients, scientists found that this blood cell had practically disappeared from the body. Without the T-cell, the body becomes incapable of destroying the many different types of infection that constantly threaten good health. In 1981, scientists could only guess the reasons why the immune systems of people with AIDS should be suppressed, or weakened, in such a way.

One suggestion at the time was that AIDS was the result of the lifestyle that some gay men led in the liberated climates of some American cities, such as San Francisco and New York. Perhaps AIDS was caused by a bad batch of 'poppers', stimulants of amyl nitrites that some gay men took to give them a high. The first report of *Pneumocystis* pneumonia in five homosexual men, published in the *Morbidity and Mortality Weekly Report* in June 1981, noted that 'all five reported using inhalant drugs'. Scientists wondered, therefore, whether this could be the cause of the new epidemic. Researchers from the Centers for Disease Control collected batches of 'poppers' to analyse – but they found nothing that could indicate why such drugs should cause AIDS although poppers did appear to suppress the immune system.

Another observation pointed to something else. Very early on in their study of AIDS, researchers from the CDC discovered that gay men who had thirty or more partners a year seemed to be far more likely to develop AIDS than gay men who had one or only a few partners. Perhaps, therefore, these more promiscuous gay men had somehow overloaded their immune systems. The theory suggested that these men were more likely to have suffered from a wide variety of sexually transmitted diseases. This constant battering of the immune system, so the idea went, meant that the T-cells became seriously 'overworked' and depleted. Doctors had noticed soon after the first few cases of AIDS appeared that gay men who had multiple partners, but without the symptoms of AIDS, had suppressed immune systems. Many had a variety of sexually transmitted diseases. Perhaps, therefore, repeated 'inoculation' of semen during sex with different men had led to the complete breakdown of the immune system, resulting finally in the infections typical of AIDS.

This theory could also apparently explain why some intravenous drug users, both men and women, were developing AIDS. These people were likely to use dirty needles and syringes, which meant that foreign particles entered the blood along with the drug. Often the drug itself was also impure. But, however plausible, the 'overload' theory could not explain why, in the summer of 1982, the CDC discovered another group of people 'at risk' of developing AIDS. These were haemophiliacs, males with an inherited disorder of the body's mechanism for clotting blood. (Female haemophiliacs are very rare.) Most haemophiliacs have to inject regular quantities of factor VIII, a substance they lack in their blood. Factor VIII is necessary for blood clots to form. Haemophiliacs who do not get factor VIII when they need it can literally bleed to death. These males did not fit into the overload theory, however. Most were neither promiscuous homosexuals nor users of illicit drugs, and some were pre-pubescent boys.

More than 350 cases of AIDS were reported in the US by the summer of 1982. A handful were haemophiliacs, none of whom had the recognizable risk factors associated with the disease. The inclusion of haemophiliacs quickly supported the idea that the disease was caused by an infective agent, probably a virus. As soon as the CDC had published the first accounts of AIDS, medical scientists suspected that a virus could be the cause of the immune suppression. The trouble was in trying to prove that any one of hundreds of viruses was the cause – and there was always the possibility that it could be a completely new virus.

The fact that haemophiliacs were now succumbing to AIDS strongly suggested that a virus was to blame. Factor VIII is made by pooling the blood serum of up to 30,000 donors and then extracting factor VIII from this pool. During the process of purification, the blood serum is filtered, which ensures that relatively large contaminants, such as bacteria and fungi, do not foul the end product. But smaller particles, such as viruses, survive. Perhaps, therefore, a virus was the cause of AIDS, and body fluids, such as semen and blood, passed it from one person to another. The CDC found that haemophiliacs with AIDS were distributed widely throughout the US, and not just concentrated in certain cities as were the homosexual sufferers. This also suggested that the infective agent was indeed lurking in batches of factor VIII sent to different parts of the US.

Further research on tracing partners of gay men with AIDS pointed to an infectious agent. The Centers for Disease Control found in 1982 that several gay men from different parts of the US had developed AIDS. They had all had sex with the same man, who also had AIDS, but not with each other. This was strong evidence that homosexuals suffering from AIDS could pass it on to other gay men. Doctors found yet more evidence that a blood-borne agent caused AIDS when they noticed that some men and women who had received blood transfusions had also developed AIDS. An infant in San Francisco had developed AIDS at the age of twenty months after receiving blood transfusions immediately following birth. The doctors traced the nineteen donors who had contributed to the batches of blood and blood products that the baby received. One of these donors had developed AIDS ten months after donating blood.

At the beginning of 1983, the Centers for Disease Control found that women who were the sexual partners of men with AIDS also developed the disease. Some of these women had become pregnant and doctors found that they had passed AIDS on to their babies. By now it was clear that AIDS was caused by an infectious agent. The exact nature of this agent was still a mystery, however.

Virologists around the world began to take an increasing interest in this strange disease. If they could discover a virus responsible for AIDS they would receive much kudos, and possibly a Nobel prize. In 1982, several scientists suggested that AIDS could be linked with known viruses. One theory was that the disease resulted from a new strain of African swine fever virus, which infects pigs. This virus was decimating the pig population in Haiti at about this time, and Haitians appeared to be yet another group at special risk of AIDS. (The risk groups seemed to have just one thing in common, the letter 'H' – homosexuals, heroin addicts, hookers, haemophiliacs and now Haitians.) The theory was that the swine fever virus had mutated and infected humans. It fitted in nicely with the knowledge that many gay men from the US spent their holidays in Haiti. Perhaps they had picked up the virus there by having sex with locals who had themselves become infected by eating contaminated pork regularly, or by having contact with infected pigs. These Americans had then taken the virus back to New York and San Francisco.

The idea also suited a grander conspiracy theory. African swine fever virus first appeared in Cuba, Haiti's neighbour, in the mid-1970s. Cuba claimed at the time that the CIA had deliberately infected the island with the virus in order to undermine the local economy, which is heavily dependent

28

on pig farming. From Cuba, this virus then spread to Haiti. Perhaps the CIA had tinkered with the virus in a way that allowed it to cross the species barrier and so infect humans as well as pigs. Could the CIA be responsible for AIDS? It was not the first nor indeed the last time that the CIA, or the KGB, was linked with the disease. For most scientists, however, the idea had little currency. Similarly, there was no evidence for the CIA or KGB having made the virus in a germ-warfare experiment that went wrong.

In 1982, the race to find the cause of AIDS had sparked the interest of a relatively small group of scientists working in a specialized area of virology. One of these scientists was Robert Gallo, then the head of a laboratory at the US's National Cancer Institute at Bethesda, Maryland. Early in 1982, Gallo and other scientists suggested that AIDS might be caused by a type of virus called a retrovirus. Usually, viruses have their genetic material in a form called DNA (deoxyribonucleic acid), just like that of humans. The viral DNA is wrapped in a coat of proteins. The virus attaches to the outer membrane of the cell it is attacking, and then injects its DNA into the cell. The cell treats the viral DNA as its own genetic material. The cell therefore uses the viral DNA as a blueprint to make viral protein. Eventually the cell manufactures vast quantities of viruses, which finally burst from the cell to infect other cells.

In the case of retroviruses, however, the genetic material is not DNA but RNA (ribonucleic acid). On its own, this type of viral RNA is next to useless, so retroviruses also have an enzyme that can make DNA from RNA. In most living things, the DNA is copied into RNA, which then goes to make proteins. In retroviruses, the sequence is RNA to DNA, then back to RNA and then to proteins. This initial reversal of the usual sequence, from RNA to DNA, explains why scientists have given these viruses the prefix 'retro'.

In 1978, Gallo and a group of scientists from Japan had both claimed discovery of the first retrovirus which infects humans. It causes a type of leukaemia, called adult T-cell leukaemia, so Gallo called this virus human T-cell leukaemia/

lymphoma virus (HTLV). (A lymphoma is a type of tumour.) In 1982, researchers in Gallo's laboratory found another retrovirus in cultured human cells, a much rarer virus that he said causes a type of leukaemia. Gallo called this virus HTLV-2, to distinguish it from the first human retrovirus, HTLV-1. In the same year, Gallo suggested that a form of the HTLVs might well be responsible for the new and devastating disease of AIDS. His reasons were these: the HTLVs attacked T-cells, they were transmitted by blood and intimate contact, and Gallo had noticed that the immune systems of some leukaemia patients infected with HTLV-1 were often suppressed. Research into another retrovirus, which causes a form of leukaemia in cats, backed up Gallo's theory. These cats also sometimes had an immune deficiency.

Gallo was not alone. In Paris, researchers at the Pasteur Institute (a research institution established in 1887 by the great microbiologist Louis Pasteur) also began to investigate the idea. One hospital in Paris, La Pitié Salpêtrière, had a patient suffering from the early symptoms of AIDS. This patient, a gay man, had a condition that doctors describe as lymphadenopathy, or swollen lymph glands. These glands, in the groin, armpits and neck, normally contain plentiful T-cells. The doctors treating this patient took a small piece of tissue from his lymph glands and, on the morning of 3 January 1983, sent it for analysis to virologists at the Pasteur Institute.

The researchers, led by Luc Montagnier, were particularly interested in patients with the early symptoms of AIDS because patients with full-blown AIDS had too few T-cells for the investigators to analyse properly. This patient offered enough T-cells to grow and to study. Montagnier's collaborators, Françoise Barré-Sinoussi and Jean-Claude Chermann, began to grow the cells in the laboratory to see whether they could spot signs of a retrovirus. Barré-Sinoussi looked for the presence of a chemical unique to these viruses, called reverse transcriptase. The procedure was a standard one. The researchers first separated the T-cells from the rest of the tissue by spinning the tissue in a centrifuge. (They then added anti-interferon, a substance capable of neutralizing the natu-

30

ral interferon in the tissue sample, because interferon seems to inhibit the growth of retroviruses.) Following this they added a chemical that stimulates the growth of T-cells, called T-cell growth factor, along with other chemical stimulants. (Gallo was one of the scientists who had discovered T-cell growth factor in the mid-1970s. He had, in the past, given the chemical to researchers at the Pasteur.)

Every three or four days, the researchers looked for viral activity. They did this by taking a sample of the culture and spinning it at high speed to concentrate any viruses as a pellet at the bottom of the test tube. They treated the pellet with a detergent, which would open the protein coat of retroviruses to release the reverse transcriptase inside – the chemical that signals the presence of a retrovirus. On 25 January 1983, the researchers at the Pasteur Institute for the first time found evidence of reverse transcriptase. On this day they had added a number of chemicals, such as RNA and the simpler chemicals that can be made into DNA, and found that molecules of DNA formed. Reverse transcriptase was indeed present: it was converting simple molecules into longer chains of DNA. This indicated for the first time that the cells from the patient were harbouring a retrovirus. Barré-Sinoussi carefully recorde₋ the event in her laboratory notebook. The activity, she wrote with the caution of an experienced scientist, was very low and so the evidence was inconclusive at this stage.

Two days later, she and Chermann looked again. The activity, measured by the amount of DNA that was made, had increased, reaching a peak on 7 February. The results looked exciting, but, on 11 February, the researchers detected that the activity had begun to fall 'which both surprised us and made us anxious', Barré-Sinoussi said later. The only other known retrovirus to infect humans at that time, Gallo's HTLV-1, had exactly the opposite effect. It caused the T-cells to multiply uncontrollably, just like a cancer, so that there is an ever-increasing amount of reverse transcriptase. This new virus seemed to be killing off the T-cells that it infected. Barré-Sinoussi later on said that 'this was our first suspicion that the virus we had was not like HTLV'. Meanwhile, Gallo and others continued to suggest that the HTLVs were the cause of AIDS.

The group at the Pasteur Institute had come across one of the peculiarities of this virus that made it so difficult to study. It grew in T-cells, but instead of causing the T-cells to multiply, so providing more fodder for the virus to infect, and thereby increasing the amount of virus to study, the virus destroyed its own habitat. Researchers had a tough time trying to produce enough virus to analyse in any detail. The French group, in those first few months of 1983, had a solution. They kept adding fresh T-cells from a healthy donor to provide a constant source of new cells within which the virus could replicate. After trying this for two weeks, Montagnier, Chermann and Barré-Sinoussi found they could increase the amount of virus they had. Furthermore, they could take small quantities of the fluid surrounding the T-cells and infect other T-cells with the virus. This showed that the virus existed outside the cells.

In virology, as in most spheres of life, seeing is believing. The French group quickly tried to photograph the virus under very high magnification. On 4 February 1983, Charles Dauguet, an electron microscopist at the Pasteur Institute, was the first person to see pictures of the virus. The images were of poor quality because the subject matter was so difficult to photograph. At the end of March and the beginning of April he took better photographs. The group from the Pasteur Institute was satisfied that the pictures were of a virus, and decided to publish the results. Before doing so, however, they wanted to see whether the virus they had found bore any resemblance to the only other known retrovirus to infect humans – HTLV (HTLV-2 was still not well known). If the French virus was not the same, then it must be a new virus. Montagnier's group asked Gallo to send samples of T-cells infected with HTLV, and also certain chemicals, called antibodies, that will bind specifically to HTLV. The body produces antibodies to fight off foreign particles. Scientists make antibodies by injecting viral proteins (in this case the proteins of HTLV) into animals. The immune systems of these animals

32

then make antibodies that attack these foreign proteins. If the virus that Montagnier's group had just found was HTLV, or even similar to this virus, then the researchers would have found that the HTLV antibodies and the new virus's own proteins would bind together like a lock and key. Virologists call this 'cross-reactivity'.

The team from the Pasteur Institute found no cross-reactions. The new virus seemed to be quite unlike HTLV. The only structural similarity appeared to be that one of the new virus's proteins was a similar size to a protein found in HTLV. How did the new virus fit in with the existing family of retroviruses? Clearly there was some link with HTLV. Both viruses were retroviruses that infected humans for a start, but how closely related were they?

Montagnier wrote a scientific paper describing these results, and sent it to the American journal *Science* for publication. *Science* asked Gallo to read the paper and make comments – it is common practice in scientific research for competing scientists to referee each other's papers before publication. Gallo was unsure whether Montagnier had really found a new retrovirus. If he had, then Gallo thought that the virus must be similar to, if not the same as, HTLV. 'Publish,' he told *Science*, but he advised Montagnier to make alterations to his paper and make it clear that his 'new' virus was closely related to HTLV. Montagnier took Gallo's advice and wrote: 'We report here the isolation of a novel retrovirus from a lymph node of a homosexual patient with multiple lymphadenopathies. The virus appears to be a member of the human T-cell leukaemia virus (HTLV) family.' The phrase would come back to haunt Montagnier. He was about to become embroiled in an ugly public row with Gallo over, among other things, the correct name for the virus. His researchers firmly believed that they had found something quite unlike HTLV. The wording of this paper gives an indication of how the scientists at the Pasteur Institute themselves seemed to be pulled in different directions. This first scientific paper to describe the AIDS virus, published on 20 May 1983, opens with the statement: 'A retrovirus *belonging* to the family of recently discovered human T-cell leukaemia viruses (HTLV), *but clearly distinct* from each previous isolate, has been isolated from a Caucasian patient with signs and symptoms that often precede the acquired immune deficiency syndrome (AIDS)' (authors' emphasis). It might seem odd that something can belong to the same family and yet be clearly distinct from all of the known members of that family. The similarity between Montagnier's new virus and Gallo's HTLV was that they were both retroviruses, and they both infected the T-cells of humans. Nevertheless, the team from Paris made it clear that they had discovered a 'novel' virus.

The French researchers did not name the new virus. They just described it as 'lymphotropic', meaning that it had an affinity for the white blood cells known as lymphocytes, the T-cells in this case. Montagnier and his team were a long way from proving that their new virus actually caused AIDS. They had, after all, only isolated it from one patient with the early signs of AIDS: 'The role of this virus in the etiology of AIDS,' they wrote, 'remains to be determined.' Nevertheless, the paper did show, for the first time, relatively clear photographs of the virus. It was undoubtably a breakthrough in the race to find the cause of AIDS.

Unfortunately for Montagnier, the scientific world virtually ignored the discovery described in his paper. One of the reasons was that three other scientific papers on AIDS dominated the same issue of *Science*. All described a link between AIDS and the HTLV virus discovered by Gallo. Two papers came out of Gallo's laboratory, and the third came from the laboratory of a close collaborator and friend of Gallo, Myron (Max) Essex of the Department of Cancer Biology at the Harvard School of Public Health in Boston. Between them, Gallo and Essex put a convincing case for the view that HTLV caused AIDS. Gallo published photographs of HTLV viruses found in an AIDS patient. He said that the patient had antibodies to HTLV proteins. He added that the relative absence of AIDS in Japan, where HTLV-1 has been prevalent for many years, may be because the people there had developed a resistance to the virus.

Montagnier's results did not fit nicely with the papers of Gallo and Essex, which became accepted wisdom. *Science* itself was unsure of the significance of Montagnier's findings. In the same issue, a reporter for the journal described Gallo's research in detail. Montagnier's work merited one sentence. *Science*, the journal that published the first description of the AIDS virus, failed to notice the true importance of the discovery. The world would have to wait a little longer to realize the importance of the French virus.

In 1987, Robert Gallo wrote of Montagnier's 'intriguing' discovery: 'The initial report . . . was hardly a conclusive identification of the cause of AIDS.' He was right. It was no good finding a virus in one patient; the team from the Pasteur Institute had to find it in many more people with AIDS, or with the early symptoms of AIDS. In the summer of 1983, Montagnier's group set about this task. The researchers concentrated on developing a test to see whether people suffering from AIDS were infected with their new virus. The aim was to compare the test results of these people with those of a control group of people not at risk of developing AIDS. If the people with AIDS were infected with the virus, but the control group was not, then the researchers were on their way to establishing a causal link between the virus and the disease.

The principle of the test was relatively straightforward. People with the virus should have antibodies to it. Therefore, if blood serum is mixed with the virus in question, or with cells containing the virus, any antibodies in the blood should identify and stick to the virus. With a few clever tricks this shows up visually – as a colour change, for example (see pp. 71–3). The problem that the group in Paris faced in the summer of 1983 was that the researchers had found it difficult to grow enough virus to make such a test. The obstacle was a familiar one: this virus quickly destroyed the cells in which it lived. The researchers had to rely on continually replenishing the T-cells in which the virus grew, a messy and unsatisfactory process.

As the French researchers came closer to a test, the administrators at the Pasteur Institute became aware of the financial benefits of developing such a blood test. The test would have to be properly patented to protect it against copying. The institute therefore deposited a sample of the new virus at France's National Collection of Cultures of Microorganisms on 15 July 1983. This is a necessary step in the patenting process. The institute, on Montagnier's advice, called the virus lymphadenopathy AIDS-associated virus (LAV), to distinguish it from other viruses, especially the HTLVs. (Later on this was abbreviated to lymphadenopathy associated virus.) Two days after making this deposition, Montagnier sent a frozen sample of the virus to Gallo's laboratory. The sample was damaged on arrival, so the team in the US failed to grow any virus from it. Gallo and his researchers were in any case preoccupied with the data they were working on showing a link between AIDS and the HTLV viruses.

Work in the laboratories of the Pasteur, meanwhile, went on at fever pitch. Barré-Sinoussi and Chermann wanted to develop a reliable test quickly and to publish their results as soon as they could. During those summer months they became convinced that their LAV was the cause of AIDS. Now they wanted to convince the sceptical world of virology as well. In September, they had their chance. More than a hundred virologists from all over the world met at Cold Spring Harbor Laboratory in New York to discuss human retroviruses. It was a closed scientific conference where reporting was not allowed. Gallo was one of the organizers, and he invited Montagnier to present his latest research.

One of the virologists at this meeting, Don Francis of the Centers for Disease Control, who listened to Montagnier's presentation, said afterwards that it was clear that the Frenchman had a totally new human retrovirus, quite unlike the HTLVs. His pictures were of a virus with a cone-shaped core. The core in the HTLVs was cylindrical. More importantly, Montagnier could now link his new virus directly to AIDS. His preliminary results with his test, he told the conference, showed that he could identify antibodies to the LAV virus in 22 of 35 patients suffering from swollen lymph glands, or

36

lymphadenopathy. He could also detect antibodies to LAV in 7 out of 40 healthy homosexual men, and antibodies in one out of 54 control samples of blood from healthy heterosexuals. Montagnier said he had 'conclusive' evidence that LAV represented a separate group of human retroviruses, quite distinct from the HTLVs.

At this stage, Montagnier's test was clearly not 100 per cent accurate. The test was most probably wrongly identifying antibodies to LAV when there were no antibodies, and failing to identify them when they were present: so-called 'false positive' and 'false negative' results. This is probably why, for instance, his test could not identify the presence of LAV in all thirty-five patients suffering from swollen lymph glands. Nevertheless, the data looked impressive. But not to Gallo. The scientific journal *Nature* later described the atmosphere following the encounter between Gallo and Montagnier: 'It seems common ground between Gallo and Montagnier that the former was unreasonably dismissive of the latter at the end of that talk; far from being applauded for his perceptiveness, Montagnier was left with the impression that he had been scorned.' Gallo still evidently believed that HTLV or a variant of it caused AIDS. The name of the book of papers from the conference at Cold Spring Harbor reflected this: *Human T-Cell Leukaemia/Lymphoma Virus, the family of human T-lymphotropic retroviruses: Their role in malignancies and association with AIDS*. The book still labelled LAV as belonging to the family of HTLVs. Gallo and Max Essex were co-editors.

During the meeting at Cold Spring Harbor, Montagnier – despite his hurt feelings – agreed to give Gallo a second sample of LAV. He did so on 23 September 1983, a week after the Pasteur Institute filed for a patent in Britain. Montagnier made one of Gallo's researchers, Mika Popovic, sign a statement promising that Gallo and his group would not use the virus for commercial gain. The sample of virus was for research purposes only. In the event, according to Gallo, the virus from Paris refused to grow in sufficient quantities to be of any good,

37

and so was useless. As events unfolded, the Pasteur Institute would later begin to doubt this version of events.

At the end of September 1983, Robert Gallo seemed to become less convinced that he was really on the right track with HTLVs. He wrote to a colleague in West Germany, Professor Freidrich Deinhardt, a leading virologist from the Max von Pettenkofer Institute in Munich, to voice his opinions, and, more importantly, for Deinhardt to pass on these thoughts to other virologists in Europe.

'Dear Fritz,' Gallo wrote:

After a recent trip to Europe I have become concerned that some people are under the impression that I believe AIDS is caused by HTLV. I am writing to you because of your central position in viral oncology [the study of cancer] in Europe, and I hope you will help me to dispel this impression when it comes up. My opinion is simply this: of the known candidates, it's a pretty good one based on conceptual grounds. When it comes to data proving the point, the results are stimulating for more studies, but clearly not definitive for any one virus . . . In my opinion an HTLV variant is the most likely candidate, and if it isn't this, it is an as yet unknown virus.

Gallo went on to describe research showing that HTLV appears to cause immune suppression. He then commented on the work of Luc Montagnier, whose latest research he had listened to just a fortnight previously, and whose virus was now sitting in a freezer in his laboratory: 'I have never seen the virus that Luc Montagnier has described, and I suspect he might have a mixture of two. On the other hand, some of his data are interesting but still far from definitive.' Even though Gallo was not now committing himself fully to the idea that HTLV caused AIDS, he was equally convinced that Montagnier was barking up the wrong tree.

The researchers in Gallo's laboratory faced the same problem as the team in Paris: all attempts to grow the virus in sufficient quantities for analysis were thwarted because the virus killed the cells in which it lived. Then, in early

November, Mika Popovic in Gallo's laboratory made a remarkable breakthrough. He tried to grow the virus in a certain strain of T-cells that scientists had discovered in 1979. Rather than killing the T-cells, the virus replicated and the T-cells multiplied continuously. This strain was called HUT-78, and the particular subgroup that Popovic used was called H9. The effect of infecting this strain of lymphocyte was exciting. Suddenly, Gallo and his researchers could begin to harvest huge amounts of the virus that they suspected might cause AIDS. They had little problem then with developing a rudimentary test to see whether they could directly link the virus to AIDS.

Gallo collected blood samples from many different people suffering from AIDS in order to see whether he could detect antibodies to his virus. In the autumn of 1983, other researchers also began to get closer to the cause of AIDS. In Britain, Abraham Karpas, of the University of Cambridge, had found a virus in an AIDS patient attending a local hospital. He published a short paper describing it, along with photographs of the virus taken at very high magnification. At the University of California at San Francisco, a team led by Jay Levy was also studying AIDS and had begun to find evidence of a new virus. And at the Centers for Disease Control, Paul Feorino and co-workers were also on the trail of isolating the AIDS virus. Gallo's team had to work fast to avoid being pipped at the post by other scientists. They knew that finding a virus was one thing, but proving that it caused the disease was another matter entirely.

At another closed scientific conference, this time held at Park City in Utah in early 1984, Jean-Claude Chermann from Montagnier's team gave more details of LAV. Gallo was also present. Chermann believed that his data must surely vindicate the belief that LAV was the cause of AIDS. After his presentation, some scientists agreed with Chermann that they had now seen conclusive evidence that LAV caused AIDS. Within a few weeks of the meeting at Park City, Gallo called Don Francis, then the head of the virology section of the AIDS programme at the Centers for Disease Control, to tell him that

39

he had also found a virus. Francis immediately wanted to compare Gallo's new virus with LAV. To do this, Francis wanted to test several hundred blood samples taken from people either developing AIDS or with full-blown AIDS to see whether they contained antibodies to either Montagnier's virus or to Gallo's virus. These results would then be compared against blood from a group of people without AIDS, and not at risk of the disease – the control group. It would be the most definitive test to discover whether science could link either, or indeed both, of these viruses to AIDS.

Francis wanted Gallo and Montagnier to use their respective viruses to test the first batch of blood samples from the CDC, and for the CDC to use both viruses for its own confirmation. At this point, however, cooperation broke down before the study could be completed properly. Francis said later that he detected a growing feeling of antagonism from Gallo. The results of this partial study were never published in full. Gallo was instead concentrating on publishing his own results. In April, news of a 'variant' of HTLV began to leak to the American press. An article appeared in the *Wall Street Journal*, followed by the *Washington Post* and the *San Francisco Chronicle*. Soon after these reports, *New Scientist* in Britain reported that Gallo had found a 'third variant' of the HTLV family. The story came from a freelance journalist who had interviewed Gallo.

On 23 April 1984, before Gallo had the chance to publish his research in the normal way – in the scientific journals – the US Department of Health and Human Services, the ultimate paymaster for Gallo's laboratory, decided to hold a press conference in Washington DC to announce the 'discovery' of the AIDS virus. The same morning, lawyers from the US government filed a patent on a test for antibodies to the virus, developed by Gallo. Margaret Heckler, then the Secretary of the US Department of Health and Human Services, took charge of the press conference, despite her sore throat. 'First,' she said, 'the probable cause of AIDS has been found – a variant of a known human cancer virus, called HTLV-3.' (It is true that HTLV-1 and 2 are both cancer viruses, but it is now known that the AIDS virus is not a cancer virus.) 'In particular, credit must go to our eminent Dr Robert Gallo,' Heckler continued, 'who directed the research that produced this discovery.' A statement from the US government cultivated the chauvinistic tone of the press conference: 'Today, we add another miracle to the long honour roll of American medicine and science.'

Gallo thanked the other members of his group for their part in the discovery of the new virus. The only time that Montagnier's work was mentioned was when reporters asked about how Gallo's HTLV-3 compared with LAV. Gallo replied: 'If it [the virus] turns out to be the same I certainly will say so and I will say so in a collaboration [sic].' He added: 'I think the two laboratories are very likely to come together although I cannot say at this point whether the two viruses are identical.'

A few weeks later, on 4 May 1984, the full details of Gallo's research emerged in Science. Gallo described how he could produce the virus in massive quantities in the H9 cells. He claimed to have identified the presence of the virus in 48 out of 167 people at risk of AIDS, but found no evidence of the virus in 115 healthy heterosexuals. It was the most convincing evidence yet published that a single virus was the cause of AIDS. Gallo, as Heckler said at the press conference earlier, named his new virus human T-cell leukaemia virus type-3 – HTLV-3. He evidently believed that the virus belonged to his own family of human retroviruses. In the eyes of the American media, Gallo was the discoverer of the AIDS virus. In Paris, however, the Pasteur Institute would soon try to convince the world that the claim to the discovery belonged to Montagnier.

Chapter 4

BATTLE FOR CREDIT

On 15 May 1984, soon after Robert Gallo published the research showing that his HTLV-3 caused AIDS, two scientists, Fred Murphy and Jim Curran from the Centers for Disease Control, went to visit him at his laboratory in Bethesda, Maryland. The CDC wanted, among other things, to establish the relationship between the French virus, LAV, and HTLV-3. The CDC had a problem on its hands. There now seemed to be two causes of AIDS, the virus that Gallo had just announced, and the virus that Montagnier had discovered a year earlier. Murphy and Curran wanted an agreement with Gallo that would allow the CDC to experiment with samples of HTLV-3. They already had samples of LAV from Luc Montagnier's laboratory in Paris.

In a memo to his boss written a month later, Murphy described the meeting, which took place in Gallo's office. Gallo had a document that he wanted the two CDC scientists to sign before they took samples of HTLV-3 away with them.

As Jim and I have stated, it was a tense moment, fraught with the possibility of non-delivery. Our tack, stated orally in several different ways as we discussed the matter with Dr Gallo, was that public-health purposes were paramount. Dr Gallo agreed. In our conversation, it became clear that comparison of his HTLV-3 prototype with the French prototype LAV occupied a separate niche – the

42

comparison was seen as having both academic and public-health purposes. Because of the latter, I offered, using several tacks, to have certain comparative tests between his HTLV-3 and the French LAV done at CDC; Dr Gallo declined each time, stating that such work would be done in his lab. It was clear from our discussion that this was the only subject which engendered such difficulty – when we switched to other themes . . . there was no problem.

The written agreement that Gallo wanted seemed to be a standard one, except for a 'seventh item', according to Murphy, which appeared to be 'for CDC only'. Gallo had given collaborators in other laboratories samples of HTLV-3, but since the CDC could be considered to be a competitor, Gallo told Murphy, a restriction would have to be placed on the use made of his virus. 'The [seventh] item stated that CDC was prohibited from using the material from [Gallo] for comparison with other viruses (taken to mean LAV or surrogate for it),' Murphy wrote in his memo. Gallo told Murphy and Curran that he was putting this restriction on the use of HTLV-3 so that his own researchers could capitalize on their basic discoveries.

Everyone now wanted to know the relationship between LAV and HTLV-3. The scientific community was confused with the notion that two viruses, with two different names, could cause the same disease. Did they both cause AIDS? Were they the same virus? In the CDC's preliminary studies of about two hundred blood samples, using primitive blood tests for antibodies to LAV and to HTLV-3, the CDC had little doubt that they were the same virus. But detailed proof, by analysing the molecular structure of the two viruses, had yet to emerge. Such analysis took time to do well.

It is possible to compare viruses in a number of ways – looking to see if antibodies match up is one way, but this only gives a crude measure of how related two viruses are. A more accurate method is to search for the presence of particular sites along the virus's genetic material, or DNA. Scientists do this by adding a number of different chemicals to the DNA. These chemicals, called restriction enzymes, cut the DNA only when the enzyme recognizes a specific site. Each type of restriction enzyme identifies a different site. The process is like snipping a necklace of beads. Imagine that each bead bears a letter from the alphabet, and that the beads are arranged in a random sequence: some restriction enzymes cut the necklace only between beads bearing the letters E and P, say, and others only between other pairs of letters. After subjecting the 'alphabet necklace' to a range of restriction enzymes, you will end up with a number of smaller segments of the necklace of differing lengths. If the sequences of letters on the beads of two necklaces are very similar or identical to begin with, then batches of the smaller necklaces that you end up with will also be similar. If the sequences of two necklaces are different, then so are the final batches of smaller necklaces (see figure 1).

The DNA of viruses (and remember that retroviruses, such as the AIDS virus, make a DNA copy of their RNA, and scientists prefer to analyse retroviruses by studying the viral DNA rather than viral RNA) is like a necklace of beads. Mix the chain of viral DNA with a number of different restriction enzymes, and you end up with a group of smaller strands of DNA, of differing lengths. If the sequences of two chains of viral DNA are very similar, or identical – showing that the two viruses are the same – then you end up with two very similar or identical groups of smaller chains of DNA. Molecular biologists call this 'restriction mapping', and it is a relatively quick way of seeing how related two viruses are.

The problem with restriction mapping is that it does not tell you anything about what is between the particular sites along the DNA that the restriction enzyme identifies. If you have an enzyme that identifies only E and P, what about the other twenty-four letters that may be in the 'alphabet necklace' between Es and Ps? It is possible for scientists to work out the detailed sequence of DNA, in the same way that it would be possible to take one bead after another from our necklace and make a note of its letter. This takes much longer than restriction mapping, but 'molecular sequencing', as the process is called, is a definitive method of identifying the

44

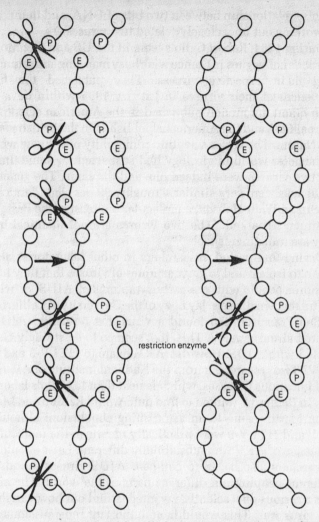

restriction enzyme

Figure 1. *Special chemicals called restriction enzymes cut the genetic material of the virus at certain sites, labelled P and E here. The sites may or may not be present, depending on the strain of the virus. Different strains therefore produce different lengths of genetic material after the treatment, which is called restriction mapping. In other words, different strains of virus have different restriction maps.*

precise relationship between two bits of DNA, and therefore of working out how closely related two viruses are.

During 1984, Robert Gallo's team in the US and Luc Montagnier's colleagues in France were busy mapping and sequencing their respective viruses. They published the full sequences of their viruses in January 1985 within days of each other: the French published in the American scientific journal *Cell*, and the Americans published in the British journal *Nature*. The wider scientific community now knew what the smaller world of virology had suspected for some time: the two viruses were indeed one and the same. The genetic sequences were very similar – roughly 99 per cent identical. As Simon Wain-Hobson, a molecular biologist at the Pasteur Institute, remarked: 'The two viruses are not identical but they are indistinguishable.'

During that period, researchers in other laboratories also began to isolate and to grow samples of viruses that they had found in people with the early symptoms of AIDS, or with the full-blown disease. Jay Levy of the University of California at San Francisco had found a virus that he called AIDS-related virus, or ARV. This, too, seemed to be strongly connected with AIDS. How did ARV relate to HTLV-3 and to LAV? Two researchers from the National Institute of Allergy and Infectious Diseases, which is next door to Gallo's laboratory in Bethesda, wanted to find out. Arnold Rabson and Malcolm Martin came to an astonishing conclusion: although LAV and HTLV-3 were practically identical, the molecular sequence of ARV was substantially different. Later on, other researchers also began to compare AIDS viruses found in different people from different parts of the world. The aim was a serious one: scientists wanted to find out how variable the virus was. This would have important repercussions in the fight to develop a vaccine. The more the virus varied, the harder it would be to make a vaccine.

Researchers from the Pasteur Institute also compared their LAV with HTLV-3, as well as with the ARV virus from California, and with two viruses found in people living in Zaïre in Africa. The chemical sequences of LAV and HTLV-3 differed by about 1 or 2 per cent. This compared to differences of about 10 or 20 per cent or more with the other three viruses. The similarity of LAV and HTLV-3 appeared to be a fluke. The AIDS virus was much more variable than the two molecular sequences of LAV and HTLV-3, published in January 1985, first suggested. Researchers soon realized that it was not going to be easy to develop a vaccine that would protect people against all the different variants of this virus.

Scientists now know that the virus that causes AIDS is quite peculiar in the extent to which it can vary – in other words, the rate at which it can mutate. In 1987, researchers at the Los Alamos National Laboratory in the US analysed the mutation rates of seventeen different AIDS viruses. They came to the conclusion that parts of the virus, for example the outer coating of the virus, called the envelope protein, may be changing at a rate five times faster than that of the influenza virus. These scientists predicted that the structure of each AIDS virus is changing overall by as much as 1 per cent a year. This means that there may be a 2 per cent difference between two viruses a year after they came from a common ancestor. Parts of the virus, such as the outer envelope protein, can change by more than 30 per cent in a short period of time. One of the scientists from Los Alamos, Gerald Myers, said that the variation of the virus that researchers first began to detect in 1985 was not the complete story: 'It became clear that what we saw in 1985 in terms of variation was only the tip of the iceberg.'

One suggestion to account for this variation relates to the enzyme reverse transcriptase, which copies the virus's genetic material, its RNA, into the other type of genetic material, DNA. This enzyme is said to be 'unfaithful'. It does not make a perfect copy of DNA from RNA all the time. Every now and again, the enzyme lets a little error slip in. In other words, it is permitting the virus to mutate, and mutations cause changes in the structure of the virus. In terms of the analogy of the alphabet necklace, it means that the reverse transcriptase is slipping in one letter when it should be inserting another into the sequence of chemicals. For a retrovirus, var-

47

iety is not just the spice of life, it is the key to survival, because it means that the virus can adapt quickly to a changing environment. For a virus such as the AIDS virus which attacks the body's immune system this is a great advantage. Its rapid rate of mutation means that the virus can continually fool the body's immune system.

The discovery of the variation of the AIDS virus began to fuel deep suspicions within the Pasteur Institute about the extraordinary similarity of Gallo's HTLV-3 and Montagnier's LAV. Could Gallo have used samples of Montagnier's virus, which Montagnier gave to Gallo twice in 1983, in order to help to make his own discovery of HTLV-3? If this was the case, then the blood test for antibodies to the virus that Gallo's laboratory had developed using HTLV-3 would represent a commercial use of the French virus. The written agreement between the Pasteur Institute and Gallo's laboratory had expressly forbidden this.

The Pasteur Institute applied for a patent in the US on Montagnier's blood test in December 1983. The US government applied for a patent on Gallo's blood test in April the following year. However, in May 1985, the US Patent and Trademark Office awarded a patent on Gallo's test, without making an award for Montagnier's earlier patent application.

The frustration felt by the scientists at the Pasteur Institute over what they believed was a failure to recognize their pioneering work eventually turned into an ugly public row involving armies of high-powered lawyers. In December 1985, the Pasteur Institute went to court. The institute wanted recognition for its scientists, and a share of the royalties that the US government was beginning to receive on the blood test developed by Gallo. Case number 730-85-C in the US Claims Court – the Pasteur Institute versus the US government – concerned one very important allegation. 'Upon information and belief,' the Pasteur's lawyers claimed, the virus at the heart of the blood test developed by Gallo 'is, or is substantially identical to, the LAV strain first isolated by Pasteur'.

Before the dispute had got this far, Gallo had tried to

explain how his HTLV-3 could be so similar to Montagnier's LAV. It might be, he said in a letter to the journal *Nature*, 'because the individuals from whom these isolates were derived acquired the virus at a similar time and place. In fact, many of our earliest HTLV-3 isolates were all from specimens obtained in late 1982 or early 1983 from the east coast of the United States, and LAV, although isolated from a Frenchman with a lymphadenopathy syndrome, had his contact in New York in the same period.'

In fact, the last time the Frenchman in question had visited New York was in 1979 – two to three years before the blood samples in question were taken from gay men, and then sent to Gallo's laboratory. Gallo implied that the similarity of HTLV-3 with LAV was because his virus had come from a sexual partner of the Frenchman who was the source of the Pasteur's LAV. This was why the two viruses were virtually identical.

The explanation had one problem, which only became apparent later on: as already mentioned, the virus mutates very quickly. Even if Gallo's blood samples had come from a sexual partner of the Frenchman, the chances are that the virus would have changed quite considerably in two to three years. At the end of 1985, nearly a year after Gallo had offered this explanation for the similarity of the viruses, a team of scientists, led by Steven Benn and Rosamond Rutledge of the US National Institute of Allergy and Infectious Diseases in Maryland, published an analysis of twelve different AIDS viruses, including LAV and HTLV-3, along with five different isolates of the virus taken from people living in New York. They subjected the viruses to seven different restriction enzymes, which were known to cleave the viral DNA at different points. They found: 'With the exception of LAV and HTLV-3, all of the isolates were different.' They also discovered that the five viruses from New York were all different from each other, and different to LAV and HTLV-3. It seemed, therefore, that the AIDS virus varied even within the same city. This did not fit well with Gallo's theory explaining why HTLV-3 was so similar to LAV.

The lawyers working for the Pasteur Institute, Townley and Updike, were eager to pounce on all this circumstantial evidence to show that Gallo's virus 'is, or is substantially identical to, the LAV strain' of Montagnier's group. The firm, which operates from offices occupying several floors of the Chrysler Building in New York City, had put a bright young lawyer, Jim Swire, on to the case. His brief was to dissect the difficult subject of virology and present the Pasteur Institute's case in plain and simple English. He was also Townley and Updike's tough guy, appointed to cope with the experienced and shrewd lawyers working for the US government. Swire once described himself as 'the hired gun' of Townley and Updike.

One of Swire's first tasks was to apply for documents from Gallo's laboratory under the US Freedom of Information laws. He wanted to know anything and everything that went on in Gallo's laboratory before and after Gallo announced the discovery of HTLV-3. He also obtained documents from other laboratories that had contacts with Gallo's lab. One of these was the electron microscopy laboratory of the Frederick Cancer Research Facility in Maryland. This laboratory took high-magnification photographs, called electron micrographs, for Gallo's researchers, who did not have an electron microscope of their own.

Swire came across a letter from the head of the electron microscopy laboratory, Matthew Gonda, to Mika Popovic, the researcher in Gallo's laboratory who first successfully grew HTLV-3. The letter, dated 14 December 1983, contained the results of analysing thirty-three samples of blood that Popovic had sent to Gonda. The letter said that just two of these samples proved to be positive for 'lentivirus' (lentiviruses are a type of retrovirus, and the AIDS virus belongs to this group).

This was a clear sign that Popovic had found the AIDS virus, and was growing it in culture. What interested Swire, however, was that Gonda had referred to each of these samples as 'LAV', because this is how these two samples were labelled when they reached his laboratory. Swire suspected that Gallo's laboratory was growing the French virus, LAV, even though Gallo had vehemently stated that the sample of

LAV he received from the Pasteur Institute failed to be of any use. Gallo says that at this time there was no other name for the AIDS virus but LAV. It was hardly surprising, he said, that his researchers labelled the virus 'LAV'.

Swire's suspicions were aroused further when he received an anonymous tip-off about an illustration that Gallo published in one of his papers describing the discovery of HTLV-3. This illustration comprised three rows of three photographs — nine pictures in all. Each row of three pictures depicted one of the three HTLV viruses in different stages of development: HTLV-1, HTLV-2, and the AIDS virus, HTLV-3. And this same photograph was distributed to reporters at the press conference to announce HTLV-3. Gallo wanted to show the similarity of HTLV-3 to the other two viruses. Unfortunately, the virus in the photographs was in fact the French virus, LAV. There had been a dreadful mistake. Somehow, the samples that Gonda took pictures of contained LAV and not Gallo's HTLV-3. Two years after Gallo first published these photographs, he had to correct his error by writing a letter to the American journal *Science*, which had first published the pictures.

Gallo later said in an interview in *New York Native*, a gay newspaper, that the mistake was a 'sloppy, embarrassing mess'. An article by one of *Science*'s own reporters said that Gallo's correction was likely to 'raise a few eyebrows. It could also have some legal ramifications.' Jim Swire, acting for the Pasteur Institute, would try to make sure of this. The mistake over the photograph came to the forefront of the legal battle. The hired gun of Townley and Updike had fired his first shot.

A central issue in the dispute between the Pasteur Institute and the US government was whether Gallo's researchers had used the French virus in order to help them to find the AIDS virus. Could it be that the sample of the French virus, LAV, somehow contaminated the virus discovered by Gallo, called HTLV-3? Gallo has always denied this publicly, and his researcher, Mika Popovic, stated that the culturing of HTLV-3 'was almost entirely confined to the tissue culture room

6B03A where *no LAV was ever used*' (Popovic's emphasis). (Contamination can and does occasionally occur in virology when a virus, say on the end of a pipette or circulating in droplets of water in the air, gets into scientists' culture media without their knowledge.)

The French, however, were suspicious of Popovic's method of growing the virus. Popovic performed an unusual step in the isolation of HTLV-3. He pooled blood sera from ten AIDS patients and inoculated a particular strain of T-cells with this pool. Virologists usually take great care to keep their sera as pure as possible when they are trying to isolate a virus. Popovic nevertheless maintained that his method increased the chances of infecting the T-cells. Some virologists say this method was a stroke of genius on the part of Popovic – which ultimately proved to be successful.

Contamination is a dirty word to virologists. It continually threatens their research results, as well as their professional reputation. Gallo knows how embarrassing contamination can be. In 1975, he published a research paper announcing the discovery of a new human virus, which he called HL23. He suggested that this virus was involved with leukaemia. A year later, other researchers showed that the HL23 'virus' was in fact a cocktail of three ape viruses: gibbon-ape virus, simian sarcoma virus and baboon endogenous virus. HL23 was apparently the product of laboratory contamination. Gallo has described this example of contamination as 'bizarre' and has hinted that he was the victim of professional rivalry that led to sabotage. 'I mean, what could it be but sabotage? One contamination can occur, but three? In fifteen years I had had one contamination from a mouse. But three?' he later told a reporter for the *Washington Post*.

Other AIDS researchers have also had to confront the possibility of laboratory contamination. Max Essex and Phyllis Kanki, of the Harvard School of Public Health in Boston, announced in 1986 that they had found a quite different strain of the AIDS virus in people living in west Africa. The virus was so different that it warranted a new name, so they called it HTLV-4. When other researchers sequenced the genetic structure of this virus they found that it was practically identical to an AIDS-like virus that infects two species of monkeys, the rhesus macaque monkey and the African green monkey. These researchers suggested that either one virus could infect three different species, which is highly unusual, or that there had been a mix-up in the laboratory and one was being confused with another. In 1988, Essex and Kanki finally admitted that there was a mix-up. One of the monkey viruses had contaminated the cultures containing human cells, which led Essex and his group to believe that they had found 'HTLV-4' (see pp. 227–30).

One of the more confusing aspects of the AIDS story is the abundance of names that scientists have given to the 'AIDS virus'. Strictly speaking, the virus should not be called the AIDS virus. The virus does not directly cause the range of diseases seen in people who are diagnosed as having AIDS. Instead, the virus causes a breakdown in the immune system so that the body eventually becomes vulnerable to a whole range of 'opportunistic' infections.

Scientists, therefore, did not want to call the virus simply the 'AIDS virus'. The name that Gallo had originally given for the virus, human T-cell leukaemia virus type 3, or HTLV-3, eventually became human T-cell lymphotropic virus type 3. Gallo decided to change the name of his virus because it was clear that the AIDS virus did not cause leukaemia, like the other HTLVs. Nevertheless, it did have an affinity, or a tropism, for T-cells, hence the change to lymphotropic. And this still meant that Gallo could call the virus HTLV-3.

However, virologists were not at all sure that the AIDS virus should be classified alongside the HTLVs, which after all were cancer viruses. There are three distinct classes of retroviruses: cancer viruses like the leukaemia viruses, a group called the foamy retroviruses and, finally, the lentiviruses, which included retroviruses that infected sheep, goats and horses. Where in all this did the AIDS virus fit in? Even when Gonda first took pictures of LAV/HTLV-3, he called it a lentivirus; evidently because under a microscope it looked so much like one.

After Gallo announced his discovery of HTLV-3 in May 1984, the bulk of the press referred to the virus under this name. During 1985, however, virologists around the world were increasingly convinced that this was the wrong name for the AIDS virus. In May 1986, an international committee of virologists suggested a more appropriate name for the virus. The committee called it the human immunodeficiency virus or HIV. From then on, the virus that results in AIDS was called HIV. (The committee gave the AIDS-like virus that researchers had found in monkeys a similar name: simian immunodeficiency virus, or SIV.) Two members of the thirteen-strong committee disagreed, however. As far as Robert Gallo and Max Essex were concerned, the correct name for the virus was HTLV-3, and they both continued for some time to call the virus by this name.

Essex claimed to have found 'HTLV-4' in west African prostitutes at about the same time that Luc Montagnier, working with some Portuguese doctors, also found a virus that caused AIDS in west Africans. This virus appeared to be structurally quite different from his first virus. For instance, the antibodies of this new virus did not react strongly with the LAV/HTLV-3 virus, now called HIV-1. Montagnier therefore called this new virus HIV-2, denoting that it was a member of the same family of human immunodeficiency viruses, but that it was sufficiently different to warrant a distinct name.

When Montagnier and his colleagues were able to look at the detailed structure of this second AIDS virus they found something quite extraordinary: the first virus, HIV-1, shared just 42 per cent of its genetic structure with HIV-2. In other words the two viruses, which both caused AIDS in humans, were not very similar to each other at all. Clearly the two viruses had evolved from a common ancestor many years ago. The question was, when did this common ancestor exist?

Back on the twenty-sixth floor of the Chrysler Building in New York City, Jim Swire of Townley and Updike was contemplating a similar question concerning common ancestors to the two viruses discovered by Montagnier and Gallo. In May of 1986, the same month that the AIDS virus was officially christened HIV, Swire won a notable success in his bid to defend the Pasteur Institute's claim on the patent on the blood test for antibodies to the AIDS virus. The US Patent and Trademark Office, which had originally decided that the US government had the rights to the patent on a test developed by Gallo, now changed its mind: it decided to make the Pasteur Institute the 'senior party' in the patent claim. This meant that the US government, and Gallo, had to justify why they thought they should have rights to the patent in preference to the Pasteur Institute.

That month was not a happy one for Gallo. Virologists around the world began to call his virus by a name he did not like, and now the onus was on him to prove that he had the claim to the patent on his blood test. On top of this he had recently published an embarrassing correction to photographs his researchers had labelled wrongly, and he knew that other people, such as Jim Swire, were trying to make capital out of his error. Added to all this, the lawyers for the US government wanted detailed and time-consuming briefings from Gallo in order to prepare their case for what had now developed into a complex web of litigation. Gallo found that he was spending as much time on this as on his research.

There were in fact three simultaneous legal disputes between the Pasteur Institute and the US government. The first case concerned whether Gallo's laboratory had breached a contract with the Pasteur Institute not to use Montagnier's sample of LAV for commercial or industrial gain. The courts had originally decided that the letter limiting the use of LAV for research purposes only, and preventing its use for commercial gain, which Mika Popovic signed, did not constitute a 'government procurement contract', which had legal standing. The Pasteur later appealed against this ruling. (The appeal was still pending when it was overtaken by other events.) The second dispute centred on the patent itself: who

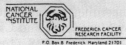

NATIONAL
CANCER
INSTITUTE
FREDERICK CANCER
RESEARCH FACILITY
P.O. Box B Frederick Maryland 21701

December 14, 1983

Dr. Mika Papovic
Laboratory of Tumor Cell Biology
NCI-NIH
Bldg. 37, Room 6B22
Bethesda, Md. 20205

Dear Mika:

Enclosed are the results of all of the samples submitted by you and members
of your lab before 12-13-83.

		Virus	Comments
1)	PB Moweni	Negative	50% degenerated cells, lymphocyte series.
2)	BM Meweni	Negative	Lymphocytes.
3)	Lg. N. Moweni	Negative	Lymphocytes.
4)	PB Yau	Negative	Lymphocytes.
5)	BM Yau	Negative	Lymphocytes.
6)	HUT 78/LAV	Positive; Lentivirus	Productive lentivirus infection with all forms of virus maturation.
7)	T 17.4/LAV	Positive; Lentivirus	Lentivirus, same comments as #6 above.

ERSELL RICHARDSON (11-03-83)

		Virus	Comments
	11-1-83 *Pool & cells*	Positive	Intercisternal A particles budding in endoplasmic reticulum. Many of the cells had degenerated.
2)	W6434 jk Da35 11-1-83	Negative	Lymphocytes.
3)	W6435 pw Da63 10-28-83	Negative	Lymphocytes.
4)	F-6357 Node Da28 10-28-83	Negative	Lymphocytes.

(PRI) PROGRAM RESOURCES, INC. • Operations and Technical Support

Figure 2. The letter from Matthew Gonda to Mika Popovic: lawyers for the Pasteur Institute claimed that the original (left) had been tampered with (right) to conceal that the French virus, LAV, was being grown.

had the rights to royalties on a blood test for antibodies to the AIDS virus? And the third court dispute revolved around the US's law on freedom of information. The US government, the ultimate employer of Gallo, had already given Jim Swire several thousand documents relating to the discovery of HTLV-3. Swire complained, however, that many of these documents arrived in a random order – deliberate obfuscation, he claimed.

It was in relation to this last court case that Swire prepared

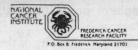

NATIONAL
CANCER
INSTITUTE

FREDERICK CANCER
RESEARCH FACILITY

P.O. Box 8, Frederick, Maryland 21701

December 14, 1983

Dr. Mika Papovic
Laboratory of Tumor Cell Biology
NCI-NIH
Bldg. 37, Room 6B22
Bethesda, Md. 20205

Dear Mika:

Enclosed are the results of all of the samples submitted by you and members
of your lab before 12-13-83.

			Virus	Comments
1)	PB	Moweni	Negative	50% degenerated cells, lymphocyte series.
2)	BM	Moweni	Negative	Lymphocytes.
3)	Lg. N.	Moweni	Negative	Lymphocytes.
4)	PB	Yau	Negative	Lymphocytes.
5)	BM	Yau	Negative	Lymphocytes.

ERSELL RICHARDSON (11-03-83)

		Virus	Comments
→ ·,	11-1-83 *Mouse* *cells*	Positive	Intercisternal A particles budding in endoplasmic reticulum. Many of the cells had degenerated.
2)	W6434 jk Da35 11-1-83	Negative	Lymphocytes.
3)	W6435 pw Da63 10-28-83	Negative	Lymphocytes.
4)	F-6367 Node Da28 10-28-83	Negative	Lymphocytes.

(PRI) PROGRAM RESOURCES, INC. • Operations and Technical Support

to fire another salvo at the US government and the lawyers representing Gallo's side of the story. Swire had uncovered not one copy of the crucial letter from Matthew Gonda to Mika Popovic regarding the photographs of virus samples (see p. 58), but two. Both copies were identical save for one thing: on one version, someone had deleted the two items referring to LAV. Instead, the letter had a rather obvious blank space (see figure 2). Interestingly, on this version of the letter, someone had scrawled a left-handed tick next to one of the blood samples that Gonda had analysed for evidence of virus particles. Swire had no idea who deleted this crucial information from the letter bearing the left-handed tick, or why. But he suspected that someone was trying to conceal the fact that

Gonda had taken good photographs of 'productive lentivirus' and that he had called it 'LAV'.

Swire prepared to present these two versions of the same letter to the US Federal Court in Washington DC as evidence that he could not rely on photocopies of documents from Gallo's laboratory. He wanted the originals. Swire was playing poker with the lawyers acting for the US government. He was trying to persuade them to settle the case out of court, and needed the help of a little gentle persuasion. He thought the two versions of the same letter would provide the necessary lubricant to settle the dispute once and for all.

Both sides were now edging towards a settlement out of court. Very senior people in both the French and the American governments began to take a keen interest in the dispute. The French government had become involved because it partly funded the Pasteur Institute. The then French Minister of Health, Michèle Barzach, had written to her counterpart in the US, Otis Bowen, in the hope of putting pressure on both sides to settle a row that had now become publicly damaging. Scientists and governments were seen to be squabbling over patents when people were dying of AIDS. It was bad for science and bad for politics. As Swire once remarked: 'This was not your usual litigation. It would be settled, if at all, at the highest levels of government.'

Towards the end of 1986, lawyers for both sides began to draw up draft documents to prepare the way for a settlement. At the same time, Gallo and Montagnier began to work out an agreed chronology of the crucial discoveries. To help them to do this, Jonas Salk, a distinguished scientist who had himself been involved in an unseemly row thirty years previously with another scientist over the polio vaccine, offered his services as mediator and umpire. Salk knew how difficult a settlement would be: 'Something like this is like an illness in science, a psychosis. Something is out of order, people take sides. The patent issue set things off, but the coin of the realm was credit, not money.'

During 1986, Montagnier and Gallo were dogged by reporters wanting to know the background to their public row. *Nature* had obtained copies of laboratory notebooks and had, according to John Maddox, the journal's editor, in a private letter to an AIDS researcher, 'embarked upon what is bound to be a complicated attempt to discover what the truth may be'.

Over Christmas 1986 and in the first few months of 1987, nearly half a dozen drafts of the settlement went back and forth between the scientists and lawyers of the two sides. During this period, however, *New Scientist* published a long article about the dispute, written by one of the authors of this book, which 'raised the temperature', according to Swire. For a short time the settlement appeared to be at risk. Both the Pasteur Institute and the US government agreed to put out an interim statement to the press condemning, without being specific, 'the inaccuracies which have appeared recently and in the past describing the dispute between the parties'. The statement added:

The parties currently are negotiating an amicable settlement which will be honourable for all. This settlement would recognize the important contributions of Dr Gallo and his colleagues and Dr Montagnier and his colleagues leading to our understanding of AIDS and its diagnosis, and such a settlement should in no way be interpreted as providing either party an advantage over the other party.

Pressure now came from the highest levels in the French and American governments to settle the dispute in time for a planned visit by the Prime Minister of France, Jacques Chirac, to the White House. Gallo flew to Frankfurt in West Germany where he met Montagnier in a hotel room to put the final touches to a settlement. 'Monty brought a bottle of cognac,' Gallo later told the *Washington Post*, 'but I told him we wouldn't drink until we'd finished.' Gallo spent his fiftieth birthday with Montagnier to work out the final wording of a chronology of AIDS research. In the same week, a letter written by some of the most eminent scientists in their field, including several Nobel prize winners, appeared in *Nature*:

We are pleased to note the approaching settlement between the United States government and the Pasteur Institute regarding patent rights related to the discovery of the human immunodeficiency virus (HIV), the virus of AIDS (acquired immune deficiency syndrome).

The letter ended:

It is important to recognize that the discovery of HIV and its relation to AIDS is only the first step towards the ultimate conquest of this disease. We need to encourage our best scientists, both young and older, to engage in solving the urgent problem posed by the spread of this virus in the human population.

On the last day of March 1987, President Ronald Reagan and Prime Minister Jacques Chirac met in the East Room of the White House to announce to the world that the dispute between the Pasteur and the US government had been settled. President Reagan said that a new foundation would be established on part of the royalties from the blood tests developed by Gallo and Montagnier. The foundation would fund research into AIDS. 'This agreement,' Reagan said, 'opens a new era in Franco-American cooperation, allowing France and the United States to join their efforts to control this terrible disease in the hopes of speeding the development of a vaccine or cure.'

The French press called the settlement between Gallo and Montagnier 'the Yalta of AIDS'. The legal document itself was forty-three pages long and was signed by twenty people, including the US Secretary for Health and Human Services, Otis Bowen, the chairman of the Pasteur Institute and Nobel prize winner, François Jacob, a number of researchers in both laboratories, and, of course, Gallo and Montagnier. In addition, Gallo and Montagnier published in Nature a long 'official' chronology of the scientific events surrounding the discovery and research into the human immunodeficiency virus. For his role as intermediary in the writing of this summary, Gallo and Montagnier thanked Jonas Salk.

60

The terms of the settlement were that the names of both Gallo and Montagnier would appear on both of their patents on blood tests for antibodies to the human immunodeficiency virus. This would circumvent the tricky issue of who had the rights to such a patent in the first place. In addition, the settlement said that 80 per cent of the royalties that accrue from the patents, from 1 January 1987 to 27 May 2002, would go to the new research foundation. The object of the foundation, the legal agreement said, was this:

The research foundation . . . shall support through grants the work of medical professionals and scientists throughout the world with respect to research into the cause, detection, prevention, treatment and cure of the disease AIDS and such other diseases caused by, or hypothesized to be caused by, a human retrovirus. The research foundation shall foster international cooperation and collaboration among medical professionals and scientists throughout the world with respect to the aforementioned research and shall also support through grants appropriate educational programmes.

Six trustees would sit on this foundation, three from the Pasteur Institute and three from the US Department of Health and Human Services. A committee of 'distinguished scientists' would assist these trustees in evaluating research proposals. A quarter of the money spent by the foundation would go towards research into AIDS in the developing world, particularly Africa.

The agreement also stipulated that each side should issue a statement to the press saying that they both disavow 'any statements, press releases, charges, allegations or other published or unpublished utterances that overtly or by inference indicated any improper, illegal, unethical or other such conduct or practice by any other Party or individual or their agents or employees.' Furthermore, clause 5 of the settlement, concerning the offical history of AIDS research published in *Nature*, stipulated:

The Parties hereto and those persons signing this Settlement Agreement in their individual capacities agree to be bound by such scientific history and further agree that they shall not make or publish any statements which would or could be construed as contradicting or compromising the integrity of the said scientific history.

In plain English, this means that neither Gallo nor Montagnier, nor anyone in their laboratories, could comment further on the events leading up to the discovery and analysis of the AIDS virus. Clause 5 did not stop President Reagan commenting on the discovery of the virus two months later during his first speech on AIDS, at the Potomac Hotel in Washington DC. 'To think, we didn't even know we had a disease until June of 1981,' Reagan told his audience, which included Gallo and Montagnier. He continued, 'the AIDS virus itself was discovered in 1984'. Reagan's speechwriters had overlooked, perhaps intentionally, that Montagnier had discovered the virus in 1983.

Nature, which had in 1986 tried to uncover the truth behind the dispute, called for the burial of hatchets. Those who want to rake over the embers of the row, editor John Maddox wrote as an oblique reference to his fellow journalists, could be likened to 'an army of ghouls'. Having presumably found the search for the truth too complicated, Maddox had now taken on the role as mediator between the two scientists. Clause 5 in the legal document would make sure that neither Montagnier nor Gallo would encourage such ghoulish behaviour. The blow-by-blow story is left for history to untangle – unless a Nobel prize committee does it first.

Chapter 5

TEST FOR INFECTION

Once scientists had found the cause of AIDS they could begin the task of designing a blood test to identify those people who might be infected with the virus. The theory is quite simple: find the virus, and then you can find the people infected with the virus. In practice, this is not quite so straightforward.

It was important to develop such a test because, by 1983, it was evident that the supply of blood to hospitals and clinics in the US during the early 1980s had been seriously contaminated with the virus. More and more people in the US who had received blood donations or products made from blood were developing AIDS. The blood supply in other countries, even if these countries did not have any cases of AIDS, had therefore also been put at risk. Many of these countries imported blood products, such as factor VIII, the blood-clotting protein, from the US. The international trade in blood and blood products had spread the virus far and wide. The trade had ensured that the virus lurking in the blood of unwitting donors had a passport to towns and cities around the globe.

Contamination of the blood supply had become a major political issue, especially in the US. When, in April 1984, Margaret Heckler, the then US Secretary of the Department of Health and Human Services, hosted the press conference in Washington DC announcing the discovery of the AIDS virus, she predicted that a test would be ready in six months and that it would be 100 per cent accurate. She was later proved wrong on both counts. The development of a commercial test took almost a year, and the test was not completely reliable.

From the outset, a 'blood test for AIDS' was fraught with technical and ethical difficulties. For a start, the test was not a test for AIDS. It was not even a test for the virus. It was a test for antibodies to the virus and as such only indicated whether somebody had at some time in the past been infected, or 'exposed', to the virus. At the time, scientists were not sure whether a positive result meant that the person was still infected with the virus, and it certainly did not automatically mean that they had AIDS, or would develop it. On top of this uncertainty, the tests that scientists were to develop during 1984 were not totally accurate; there was always a risk that the test would wrongly diagnose people as having antibodies to the virus when they did not, and, conversely, wrongly diagnose people as not having antibodies when in reality they did.

Yet another problem with the blood test stemmed from its development as a means of screening donated blood to see whether antibodies to HIV were present. The test was developed primarily in order to stop infected people from donating blood, so clearing the blood banks of the virus. The use of the test as a diagnostic tool to tell patients their antibody status was a spin-off. The test immediately created difficult ethical dilemmas for the medical authorities: should they tell blood donors if the test indicated that they were carriers of the virus, and if so what sort of counselling should be given to them and their families or lovers? After all, many people, rightly or wrongly, would see a positive test as a death sentence. It could create all kinds of emotional and psychological problems. And what if the test was wrong? What about third parties – employers, insurance companies and even medical staff looking after these people? Should they be told of positive results as well?

Such difficult questions had, however, become secondary

to the task in hand – the blood supply must be cleared of the virus. The spectacle of children and babies developing AIDS as a result of contaminated blood transfusions, or blood products such as factor VIII, had resulted in hysterical articles in the press, describing these children as 'innocent victims', with the obvious insinuation that other 'AIDS victims' were in some way 'guilty'. The public's anxiety was aroused. No longer was AIDS a disease of gays and drug addicts. 'Ordinary' people, anyone who needed blood, were also now at risk of what was originally thought to be the problem of the minority.

In the US, this anxiety began to spread to the political establishment – 1984 was an election year for President Reagan, and AIDS, especially a blood supply that was contaminated with the AIDS virus, had threatened to become an important election issue. Heckler, and others within the Department of Health and Human Services, wanted a blood test quickly. Almost immediately after Robert Gallo had claimed the discovery of the AIDS virus, 'HTLV-3' as he called it at the time, the health department launched its own campaign to develop a test that could detect antibodies to the virus. The department invited American drug companies to tender for licences to manufacture such a test, based on Gallo's HTLV-3 and the type of blood cell in which it appeared to thrive, the H9 line of white blood cells. Twenty companies took up the challenge. They knew that they could make millions of dollars from selling the test kits to blood banks and other organizations wishing to screen people for the virus. The US government was itself interested in screening people wanting to enter the military services. The potential world market for a 'test for AIDS' was enormous.

The US health department eventually gave licences to develop a blood test to five companies. These were Abbott Laboratories, from Chicago, Electro-Nucleonics from Maryland, Du Pont of Delaware collaborating with Biotech Research Laboratories of Maryland, Litton Bionetics also of Maryland, and Travenol Genentech Diagnostics of Cambridge, Massachusetts. The health department gave each company twenty-five litres of H9 cells infected with Gallo's HTLV-3, the AIDS virus, in June 1984. The race had begun to develop a test to rid the US blood supply of the virus.

At this time, the blood supply in the US and elsewhere remained open to contamination with the AIDS virus. As early as the spring of 1983, the medical authorities in the US had urged people not to give blood if they were in any of the high-risk groups for AIDS. European governments, including those of Britain and France, made similar requests. However, many people were afraid that closet gays and other people with a habit or lifestyle they had kept to themselves would continue to give blood because not to do so after being a regular donor might expose them in the eyes of their friends and families. Of course, blood banks could ask donors about their lifestyle in a confidential questionnaire, but this would not guarantee that those at risk of being infected with the virus would refrain from giving blood.

In the period immediately after Gallo announced the discovery of HTLV-3, the medical authorities in the US were in a strange and difficult position. The cause of AIDS had apparently been found, and yet the authorities were seemingly helpless to prevent contamination of blood. Apart from urging high-risk groups not to donate blood, the only alternative precaution was a complete ban on the collection and sale of blood and blood products. This was not a viable option. It might be risky to receive donated blood, but it would be far riskier for most patients not to have blood transfusions at all.

There was in fact another suggestion, articulated by President Reagan in 1986: 'You know, there's a practical solution to that if someone would just announce it,' he told the *Los Angeles Times*. 'Why don't healthy and well people give blood for themselves? And then it can be kept in case they ever need a transfusion. They can get a transfusion of their own blood and they don't have to gamble . . .' This suggestion was not a new one. Doctors had considered autologous transfusions (i.e. of the patient's own blood) several years earlier, but had concluded that for the vast majority of patients it would be impractical and too difficult to organize.

Scientists, being the creatures they are, saw a unique research opportunity in the dilemma facing doctors in 1984. While they were waiting for the drug companies to develop blood tests for AIDS antibodies, they decided to conduct a study that would help them to understand more about how AIDS is transmitted. This study was to exploit the fact that some people carrying the virus would inevitably give blood and this would end up being transfused into people who might then develop AIDS. Essentially the study was to see what would happen to people years after they received blood which was later found to have contained antibodies to the AIDS virus.

The director of the US's National Heart, Lung and Blood Institution, Claude Lenfant, explained the reasons behind the study to *Science*: 'Between now and the time a test is commercially available, we have a unique scientific opportunity to learn about the transmission of this disease.' He added: 'But it is important to emphasize that this study can only take place because the blood we want to collect and screen will be used in the usual course of blood banking now whether we do our study or not. An informed-consent form must clearly explain that we are not deliberately transmitting AIDS.'

It seems that even before a blood test had become available, ethical problems over an 'AIDS test' had arisen – informed consent became the issue. An informed-consent form is a document that people sign as evidence that they not only consent to a particular type of medical treatment, but that they are also aware of what is at stake – in other words, that they are fully informed of the implications of the treatment. This particular study planned to include 200,000 normal, healthy donors who did not fall into any of the risk categories for AIDS. They were asked to consent to a sample of their blood being stored until a blood test became available some months later. Their blood, meanwhile, would be used in medical treatment in the routine way. Once the test kits were ready, these stored blood samples would be tested for antibodies to HIV. The researchers would then follow up those people who had received blood from donors who had proved positive for antibodies to HIV.

At the time that this study was proposed, there was a great deal of debate within the American medical establishment about the ethics of 'informed consent'. According to *Science*, three out of four blood banks that were to take part in the study did not want to tell blood donors that their blood was to be tested for the antibodies. It was the first portent of the ethical debates to follow. As *Science* said:

Because the first mass screening tests will be able only to detect antibody to AIDS in the blood, they will provide little clear information about whether the person is at risk of getting full-blown infection or whether he has simply been exposed to HTLV-3 and mounted a successful immune response. Heterosexual blood donors who test AIDS positive could be falsely labelled [as] homosexuals if the information leaked out. Healthy, non-promiscuous homosexuals also worry about the stigma that an AIDS-positive test would attach to them. All round, there is concern about what the information would mean to prospective employers or health-insurance companies . . . Thus, for many reasons, the likelihood that giving the donor complex, unclear, but frightening information will cause at least psychological stress is very high.

Another argument against telling a blood donor about a positive result was that this would attract to the blood banks the very people that blood banks did not want. Some homosexuals and drug users would, no doubt, donate blood in the hope that they would have a blood test for AIDS and so find out about their antibody status. The medical authorities in Britain, and later in the US and elsewhere, quickly decided that any introduction of a test to screen blood for HIV at blood banks must not occur without offering, at the same time, anonymous testing at clinics for sexually transmitted diseases. In this way, people wanting to know whether they had antibodies to the AIDS virus could do so without giving blood. This evidently meant that a test that was being designed to screen donated blood was now also going to be used, for better or for worse, to 'tell' people whether or not they had been infected with HIV.

The implications of this took second place to clearing the blood supply of the virus. As *The New York Times* said: 'Blood has become the cornerstone of modern medicine, more significant to treatment than many drugs.' In the US alone, doctors administer about 12 million blood transfusions each year to about 3.5 million people. As a leading specialist in blood transfusions, Johanna Pindyck of the New York Blood Center, said in an interview with the same newspaper: 'It is a toss-up between transfusions and anaesthesia as to which has had a greater impact on surgery. You could put people to sleep and still not do the procedures that you are able to do now if it weren't for blood transfusions. Moreover the whole health care systems could not have developed without blood.'

The medical establishment clearly felt, therefore, that ridding the blood supply of the virus was a top priority. Scientists in the five companies in the US with licences to use Gallo's virus and the H9 cell line were working flat out in the summer and autumn of 1984 to develop test kits. At the same time, the American medical authorities were preparing advice for doctors, blood banks, and eventually the public in regard to the new test. The Department of Health and Human Services wrote to American physicians in February 1985 warning them that a blood test for antibodies to the AIDS virus would soon be licensed by the US Food and Drug Administration, the statutory body in the US concerned with the approval of new types of medications. 'This is NOT a test for AIDS', the letter emphasized.

The health department had decided that people should be made fully aware of what the 'AIDS test', as it was being referred to in the press, really was. Information about the significance of a positive result should be given to patients before the test takes place, the health department told American physicians: 'In addition, physicians and other health professionals should recognize the need for assuring confidentiality of test results because loss of employment or insurability may occur if positive test results become a part of the medical record,' said the department.

In its advice to the blood banks, the US health department recommended that each establishment should appoint a trained counsellor who would tell blood donors about positive results for blood tests when these occurred. The counsellors, the health department said, must 'understand the need for confidentiality and the severe psychological stress that reactive [positive] tests will cause in some individuals.' Even at this early stage in the application of a 'test for AIDS', the health authorities had a good idea of the demand that there would be from third parties to have access to the results of blood tests. 'In all cases,' the health department told blood banks, 'it will be extremely important to protect the confidentiality of donor identity in relation to test results and to restrict access to information . . . The misuse of such information could have serious consequences for both donors and blood establishments because positive test results could result in loss of employment or insurability.'

Having prepared doctors and blood banks for the impending blood test, the US Food and Drug Administration issued a licence for the sale of the first of the test kits in March 1985. The 'test for AIDS' had finally arrived.

Of course, the blood test was not a test for AIDS. It was a test for antibodies to HIV, the molecules that the body produces when infected by any microorganism. From the outset it became obvious that detecting the presence of the virus itself was too difficult for a test that would have to be cheap, accurate, sensitive and fast. Trying to establish the presence of the enzyme reverse transcriptase, which is how the scientists at the Pasteur Institute in Paris first found the virus, in millions of blood samples was just not feasible. It would be far too cumbersome and time-consuming. Far better to design a test that would detect the presence of antibodies to the virus. After all, if a person had antibodies to HIV then this meant that they had been exposed to the virus and therefore could possibly still transmit it.

Trying to detect the virus directly has other problems. The amount of HIV circulating in the bloodstream of an infected person can vary depending on the stage of infection. Even when the amount of virus is at a maximum – perhaps at the stage when AIDS is developing – there is still precious little virus to detect accurately in any one blood sample. Despite this, infected people can still pass the virus to others. There have been more recent technical advances that permit scientists to detect the virus directly (see p. 79), but in 1984 researchers felt that the best blood test would be a test for detecting antibodies to the virus. Once the body produces antibodies to a foreign particle, such as a virus, they are relatively abundant in the bloodstream, and can almost always be found there long after the initial infection has taken place.

The American companies, each working with twenty-five litres of HIV from Robert Gallo, courtesy of the US government, began to design a test based on a technique called enzyme-linked immunosorbent assay, or ELISA for short. This type of test for antibodies can exist in a number of different forms, but they all share the same basic technology. Most ELISA tests can be likened to layers in a sandwich. In the ELISA test for HIV, the first layer in the sandwich is viral proteins, which the companies purified as best they could and then attached to resin beads, or the sides of small depressions or 'wells' in a plastic dish. Scientists call these beads or wells the 'solid phase' and it means that anything sticking to this solid platform will not be washed away.

The next layer in the 'sandwich' consists of the antibodies to the virus. The virus is made of many different types of proteins (as we discuss in Chapter 7), and in the body each protein (or antigen) causes the production of a particular antibody that specifically recognizes and sticks to that protein. The companies attempted to use viral proteins that are particularly good at 'raising' antibodies. Adding a blood sample containing antibodies to the proteins attached to the solid phase causes the second layer of the sandwich to form as the antibodies latch on to the antigens.

The problem now is how to discover whether or not anti-

S. F. T. V.—5

71

bodies are stuck to the solid phase; if they are, then the blood sample has antibodies to HIV, and the test is positive. To find out, a further layer is added to the sandwich. This layer is another chemical that will bind to the antibody. It is in turn attached to a substance, called an enzyme. The final step in the test is to add a solution containing a chemical that the enzyme, if it is present, will cause to change colour.

An important feature of the ELISA test is that the solid phase is frequently washed so that anything not bound to it (either directly or in a chemical complex) is washed away. If, therefore, there are no antibodies to the virus in the blood sample, then nothing, including the enzyme, will remain after washing. Therefore there will be no change in colour – a negative result (see figure 3).

There is a slight variant of this test which does not rely on an enzyme to change the colour of the solution. This technique uses instead the phenomenon called immunofluorescence, when certain chemicals show up or 'fluoresce' when illuminated with ultraviolet light. In this test, the chemical that binds to the antibody to HIV and the 'sandwich' sitting on the solid phase contains a fluorescent dye instead of an enzyme. The presence of antibodies to HIV becomes evident when the blood sample fluoresces in this way. One of the first scientists to develop such a fluorescent test was Takeshi Kurimura of Tottori University in Japan. He had perfected his test by April 1985.

One of the first commercial tests to receive a licence from medical authorities, however, came from Abbott Laboratories and was based on the standard ELISA process. In a press statement in March 1985, Abbott claimed that its test identified forty-seven positive results in 18,000 samples of blood, 'indicating excellent specificity', the company said. (Specificity, in terms of such blood tests, is defined as the ability of a test to determine healthy people as negative for the virus. In other words, a highly specific test gives rise to a low number of false positives.) Abbott failed to mention how many of these forty-seven positive results its test had *falsely* labelled as positive. A second, back-up test is needed to make sure that

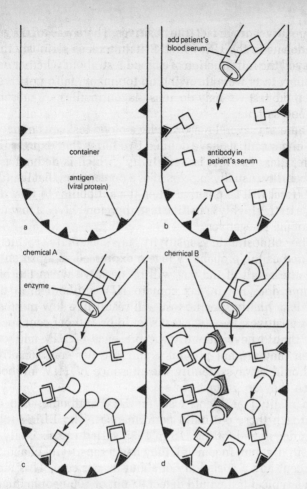

Figure 3. The standard blood test for infection with HIV is called the ELISA test. The manufacturers of this type of test supply specially prepared containers which have viral proteins, or antigens, stuck to the sides. These antigens cannot be washed off. Anything that sticks to the antigens cannot be washed away, either. If antibodies to HIV are present in the blood sample added, they stick to the antigens. When chemical A is added, it will stick to these antibodies to HIV if they are present. Only if chemical A, which incorporates an enzyme, remains behind after washing, will chemical B change colour. So, with this type of test, a colour change indicates a positive result.

the positives are in fact true positives. There was to be a growing debate in the US, which Britain took so seriously that it delayed the introduction of a blood test, about whether or not the new tests were throwing up too many 'false positives' – when the test wrongly decides that antibodies are present in a blood sample.

There are several reasons why a blood test can be inaccurate, and scientists have defined two terms that express these difficulties. The first is 'sensitivity', which is defined as the probability (usually expressed as a percentage) that the result of the test will be positive when the antibodies to HIV do in fact exist. A highly sensitive test, therefore, gives a low number of false negatives.

The opposite to sensitivity is 'specificity', which is defined as the probability (again expressed as a percentage) that the result of the test will be negative when the blood sample does not in fact contain HIV antibodies. In other words, a highly specific test will result in a low number of false positives. Ideally, a test should be 100 per cent specific – it should never identify the presence of HIV antibodies when they are not present – and 100 per cent sensitive – it should always identify the presence of HIV antibodies when they are in fact there.

In reality, the blood tests for HIV antibodies can only approach these optimum performances. The ELISA blood tests developed for the US in 1985 varied in specificity and sensitivity, but, in general, they had a sensitivity of about 97 per cent and a specificity of about 99 per cent. This means that a typical test would detect 97 out of 100 people infected with the virus, and identify as negative 99 people out of 100 who were not infected with the virus. Tiny changes in specificity can have dramatic consequences. For instance, if the true prevalence of the infection is one positive result in every 1,000 blood samples, a test which is 99.8 per cent specific will, from 1,000 samples, find one true positive and two false positives. If the test is only 99.2 per cent specific, however, it will detect one true positive and eight false positives – quite a dramatic difference.

At first glance, the relatively low sensitivity of the tests might seem a little surprising. It would appear that the blood tests miss, on average, three out of every hundred people infected with the virus. If millions of people are screened then this might mean that the test is failing to identify tens or hundreds of infected people, with catastrophic consequences for the safety of the blood supply. In fact this interpretation is wrong, because of another factor called the 'predictive value' of the blood test. The predictive value is a measure of how well the test performs in a given population and it can be applied to both a positive result and a negative result. For instance the predictive value of a positive result is the probability that the person will be infected if the result of the test is positive. Similarly, the predictive value of a negative result is the probability that a person is not infected if the result of the test is negative.

Predictive values are not fixed; they change with the prevalence of the virus in the population. If a particular virus has infected 30 per cent of the population, for instance, then the predictive value of a positive result of a test with 97 per cent sensitivity and 99 per cent specificity is nearly 98 per cent (we will not go into the mathematics of how this is calculated). And the predictive value of a negative result with the same test is nearly 99 per cent, which is pretty good.

If, however, the virus in question is not very prevalent in the population being screened, which is the case with HIV in blood donors in many developed countries (where it infects fewer than 0.1 per cent), then the predictive value of a positive result changes dramatically – it is less than 10 per cent. Meanwhile, the predictive value of a negative result increases to almost 100 per cent.

This situation may seem odd at first, but common sense says that when a test result is negative for a virus that infects fewer than 1 in every 1,000 blood donors, it is more likely to be accurate than when the virus infects, say, twenty in every hundred people. This explains why the tests in question were better at identifying true negative results in a population of blood donors where the prevalence of the virus was extremely low, than in a population of homosexual men where the prevalence was quite high.

Because of these predictive values for a population of blood donors, it was not necessary to check a result that turned out to be negative. If a result proved positive, however, it had to be checked again, preferably using another test. If this too proved positive, then a third type of test would be the final confirmation that antibodies were indeed present.

The most common type of confirmatory test is known as the Western blot. This test can be highly accurate with the correct reagents and experienced technicians. It is also, unfortunately, quite complex and therefore expensive to carry out. The Western blot works by first teasing apart all the different proteins in the virus. This is done by putting the proteins from mashed-up viruses in a semi-fluid gel and exposing them to an electric field; the proteins, which are charged particles, move at different speeds, depending on their size. After a period of time the proteins are arranged in a column with, typically, the lighter proteins, having moved further, at one end and the heavier and larger ones at the other. The proteins are then transferred in these positions to strips of nitrocellulose gel.

It is then possible to treat the viral proteins attached to the nitrocellulose similarly to the 'solid phase' in ELISA tests. Antibodies, and radioactive chemicals which stick to these antibodies, will bind to the nitrocellulose strips. It is then possible to detect the presence of the radioactive chemicals by exposing a photographic emulsion to the strip. This emulsion will darken if the chemicals are present (see figure 4). The great advantage of Western blotting is that it identifies the range of antibodies that may be present in response to the spectrum of viral proteins of human immunodeficiency virus. Researchers have suggested that once a person becomes infected with HIV and 'seroconversion' (the production of antibodies against the proteins of HIV) occurs, antibodies first appear against the gp41 protein of the viral envelope and the p24 protein of the protein core

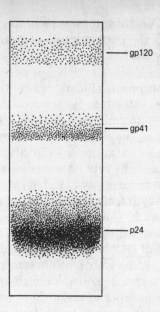

Figure 4. *The pattern of a Western blot test shows whether a person is infected with HIV. If the test is positive, dark bands appear, indicating the presence of antibodies to various viral proteins, such as p24, gp41 or gp120. The p24 band frequently shows the strongest reaction.*

of the virus (for a detailed discussion of the structure of HIV, see p. 98). Antibodies against the other proteins of HIV appear at a later stage.

Western blotting is not foolproof. False positives and false negatives do occur. However, the test looks for the presence of a range of antibodies and so, providing the laboratory technician looks for more than one antibody, the final outcome is highly likely to be an accurate result. A disadvantage of Western blots, which they do not, in general, share with other tests, is that the result relies on the skill of the technician interpreting the result. This is one of the reasons why Western blotting is carried out by research laboratories rather than commercial organizations, which may not have the skilled staff to make the correct interpretation of the visual pattern produced by the blot.

Technology is refining blood tests continually. Since the first tests became available in 1985, scientists have devised a number of different techniques to make the tests more specific and more sensitive. They have also developed tests that can detect viral proteins – the antigens – directly, rather than their antibodies. These tests rely on essentially the same principles as ELISA tests for antibodies, but this time antibodies from people already infected with HIV are used as the first layer of the 'sandwich', thus reversing the layers. The great advantage of these so-called antigen tests is that doctors can detect the presence of HIV before the person develops antibodies to the virus – in other words, before seroconversion occurs. It is difficult, however, to collect enough antibodies to HIV and purify them in order to make these tests in bulk. One way around the problem is to fuse a human antibody-producing cell with a mouse cell to create a cell that makes only the human antibody to HIV. Several companies have developed tests based on these so-called monoclonal antibodies.

Another approach to testing is to make viral antigens by inserting HIV genes into a bacterium. Grown in bulk, the bacteria make the viral proteins and these synthetic antigens can then be attached to latex beads. When a drop of infected blood is added to the beads, antibodies in the blood will cause the beads to stick together to form tiny clumps that the tester can see with the naked eye. Such 'latex agglutination' tests take minutes rather than hours to perform and are especially useful for developing countries, where there may not be the sophisticated facilities necessary for standard ELISA tests.

A variation on this is called the Karpas test, which uses a strain of human tumour cells that exhibit the trait of becoming loaded with viral particles. Infected blood causes a colour change that can be seen with the naked eye. Yet another type of '10-minute' test is made by Du Pont de Nemours and called Hivchek. Infected blood causes a red spot to appear on the test, which contains a colloidal gold substance that changes colour in the presence of antibodies to HIV. Further tests are being developed to use saliva or urine from potentially infected people. These tests will be as easy to use as do-it-yourself pregnancy tests.

The appearance of such instant and easy-to-use test kits prompted the British and the American governments to limit their use to the medical profession. In 1988, the US Food and Drug Administration issued such stringent guidelines for across-the-counter selling of home test kits that it is unlikely that any drug company would want to see approval for such marketing. In the same year, the British Department of Health added a clause to a health bill passing through Parliament which bans the unauthorized sale of kits that people could use themselves. Both governments were concerned that it would be too dangerous to allow unrestricted sale of test kits without the benefit of trained counselling and confirmatory testing.

Perhaps in anticipation of the ethical problems that its new test causes, Du Pont published its own protocol for using Hivchek in advertisements for the product. There should be a clinical reason for testing, the patient should give informed consent to the doctor, a repeat test should be made for positive results, and details of confirmed positive results should be given only to the doctor doing the diagnosis, the company said.

The most revolutionary test to have been developed in recent years is the test based on a technique for amplifying minute quantities of DNA. This allows researchers to look for the tiny amounts of DNA from derived HIV that have become incorporated into the cells of infected people. Before the amplification technique, called the polymerase chain reaction (PCR), became available, it was exceedingly difficult to locate and identify the extremely small quantities of viral DNA that hide within the masses of human DNA present in the cell.

The technique is first to synthesise a short strand of DNA that has a complementary sequence of chemical bases to part of the DNA of the virus. This 'primer' is added to the soup of viral and human DNA and its components, which is heated to separate the double strands of the molecule. The primers stick to the viral DNA hiding within the human DNA. Researchers then add a special enzyme, called a polymerase, that was found in bacteria that live in hot, natural springs. This enzyme is therefore heat resistant. The polymerase zips along the single-stranded molecule to make the double-stranded helix once more – something that all polymerases can do.

This polymerase is not destroyed by the heating that separates double-stranded DNA. Further cycles of heating and cooling do not affect the enzyme, which continues to make two strands from only one. Each cycle of heating results in the doubling of the viral DNA. Two strands become four, four become eight, eight become sixteen, and so on. In this way, scientists can make billions of copies of just one copy of viral DNA. And so, what was difficult or impossible to detect because of its small quantity, now becomes readily retrievable.

For instance, Steven Wolinksy and John Phair at the Northwestern University Medical School in Chicago, said in 1988 that PCR allows them to detect about six molecules of viral DNA in 15,000 human cells – equivalent to finding a needle in a haystack. The PCR test, as soon as it was used on certain people at risk of AIDS, revealed some startling details of the biology of HIV. Wolinksy and Phair, for example, found that the time taken between infection with the virus and development of antibodies could, in some people, be as long as several years. Up to then scientists had believed that the incubation period was no longer than about six months. In one group of homosexual men whose blood had been stored for several years before they started to prove positive with conventional antibody tests, Wolinksy and Phair detected viral DNA in the stored samples for one or two years before the men produced antibody to HIV. In one man, this period of incubation lasted three and a half years.

The PCR test is also proving invaluable for the true diagnosis of babies born of infected women. The problem until PCR came along was that an infant's antibodies to HIV could have come from the mother via the placenta. Now, it is possible to discover whether a newborn child really is infected with HIV. The full implications of the PCR test are unlikely to be realized until it is used on a wide scale. But early results of PCR testing clearly indicate that infection with HIV is a more complex process than scientists once thought.

Chapter 6

A TESTING TIME

When blood tests became available in the US, in March 1985, the British government came under pressure to introduce tests too, using the American kits if necessary. The same happened in France. Neither country, however, introduced its testing programme until nearly six months after the US had begun screening blood. Coincidentally, both France and Britain were working on their own blood tests, and did not introduce screening programmes until these tests were ready. This brought criticism that the delay was unnecessary – both countries could have used the American tests and so have saved valuable time.

In Britain, the Department of Health and Social Security was particularly sensitive to the suggestion that it had delayed the introduction of a blood test in order to give a British pharmaceuticals company, Wellcome, the time to develop its own test. In France, the test the government approved was based on the virus isolated by Luc Montagnier and his colleagues at the Pasteur Institute in Paris, and subsequently used by Diagnostics Pasteur, a French company associated with the institute. It was easy to see why some people thought that chauvinistic pride in both countries had come before national priorities.

In the summer of 1985, under constant pressure to introduce a blood test, the British Minister of Health, Kenneth

Clarke, explained the reasons for not immediately using the tests that were already being used to screen blood in the US:

I understand and share the concern to get these tests in use as soon as possible. However, we must have tests which are accurate and can be trusted. A number of test kits are already available and in use abroad but reports from these countries suggest that the tests are not entirely reliable. We believe that no test should be introduced in the UK until its reliability has been established. There is no point in introducing a test which often fails to detect antibodies in blood or detects antibodies where there are none.

This was a slap in the face for the American health authorities, who had already approved blood tests for the US's screening programme. How accurate were the kits at that time? Nobody was more interested in this than the US. In the first few months of the screening programme, the American Red Cross and other organizations concerned with collecting and distributing blood began to collate information on the number of positive results they found in the millions of blood donations they had tested. In one study, stretching from April to June 1985, and accounting for about 70 per cent of the blood supplied in the US during this period, researchers found that 0.85 per cent of the blood donations were positive for antibodies to HIV on the first test. Using a second test as a check, the number of so-called 'repeatedly reactive' samples was reduced to 0.25 per cent.

The prevalence of repeatedly reactive blood samples varied from one geographical region to another (0.14 per cent in the north-west to 0.29 per cent in the north-east of the US). Interestingly, repeatedly reactive rates were higher in females than in males – causing speculation that HIV was perhaps more prevalent in the heterosexual population than had been thought.

In fact, these figures proved inaccurate. Many of these results were false positives and some researchers commented at the time that the blood tests then being used in the US 'cannot be used to define true positives'. Nevertheless, researchers were almost unanimous in saying that the tests had made the US's blood supply safer. Better to have a few false positives than to have no mechanism at all for detecting true positives.

There are several ways in which the result of a blood test can be false. Technicians can make mistakes such as diluting the reagents too much, splashing the specimens or flooding the wells so that the liquid from one well on the test plate runs into another. False negative results can occur simply because the person concerned has not yet developed antibodies to HIV even though infection has occurred.

But perhaps the most common reason for the high rates of false positive results detected in the early American tests was the design of these tests. The proteins of HIV were stuck to the solid phase, ready to capture any antibodies in the blood samples, as we have described. Unfortunately, as HIV buds from the human cell it infects, it becomes closely associated with human proteins in the membrane of the cell. These human proteins, called cellular antigens, also become attached to the solid phase of the test kit and so ordinary antibodies, which have nothing to do with recognizing HIV, can become attached to the solid phase – so producing a false positive result.

A way round this difficulty is to use what is called a 'competitive' test. Here, the HIV proteins are bound to the solid phase in the same way as in the non-competitive test, but the difference is that the blood specimen is added at the same time as a specific, pre-prepared antibody to HIV. This antibody is also linked to an enzyme that can turn the solution a different colour (see figure 5). In this way the real antibody to HIV (if it exists in the blood sample) and the manufactured antibody compete with each other for the limited 'landing sites' on the solid phase. This means that a strong colour shows that there are no HIV antibodies in the blood sample, as all the landing sites have been occupied by the added HIV antibody, and a weak colour shows that the antibodies exist.

British researchers designed this type of 'competitive' test for HIV antibodies; a British pharmaceuticals company,

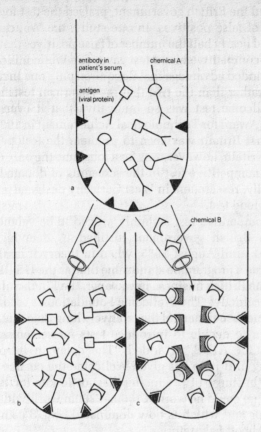

antibody in
patient's serum

chemical A

antigen
(viral protein)

a

chemical B

b

c

Figure 5. A competitive ELISA test is slightly different from the standard ELISA. Antibodies to HIV in the added blood sample compete for 'landing sites' (viral antigens on the surface of the container) with chemical A which incorporates an enzyme. If antibodies to HIV are present in the blood, few molecules of chemical A will have a chance to stick to the antigens. So chemical A will be washed away. Chemical B, however, changes colour only if chemical A is present. If chemical A has been washed away, no change in colour will occur: a positive result. If chemical A is present, chemical B will change colour: a negative result.

Wellcome, developed the design into a product. The company, and the British government, praised the test for its low number of false positives. In one study, the Wellcome test produced nearly half the number of false positives that a similar, non-competitive blood test gave. The Wellcome test also had the added advantage that it required only one incubation period, rather than the two that the American tests needed. The Wellcome test was so innovative that it even won a Queen's Award for Technological Achievement in 1987, indicating that Britain was keen to promote the test to foreign buyers. Britain, however, was for a long time the only country to use a competitive test in the screening of donated blood. Eventually, researchers in West Germany designed a similar type of blood test.

The competitive test certainly proved to be valuable, but was the British government justified in delaying blood screening until August 1985, when in theory it could have introduced a programme at the same time as the US – in April 1985? The British business newspaper, the *Financial Times*, put it succinctly: 'The Wellcome Foundation . . . is likely to be the chief beneficiary of the relatively long time that Britain has taken to decide to introduce tests for screening blood supplies for AIDS.' It added: 'The delay in introducing screening in Britain has given Wellcome the chance to leap into the business of producing diagnostic kits for AIDS, a market that could be worth £100m–£200m worldwide by the late 1980s and which is now dominated by US companies, chiefly Abbott Laboratories.'

The blood transfusion service in Britain justified the delay on the grounds that British scientists needed to evaluate the tests with British blood. As John Barbara and Patricia Hewitt, of the National Blood Transfusion Service in north London, explained in a letter to *New Scientist*: 'It would have been irresponsible not to have seen for ourselves how the various tests performed in the hands of British transfusion microbiologists and when applied to British donors.' Furthermore, there was still the problem with the high rate of false positive results observed with some American tests. Tony Napier, the medical director of the blood transfusion service in Cardiff, pointed out that these tests would wrongly label many thousands of blood donors as being HIV positive, 'donors who will require interviews, repeat tests and sympathetic counselling. And for many of these, disruption of family and social life will be unavoidable . . . The current policy regarding the introduction of testing within Britain has not been a distant bureaucratic decision.'

Less than a year after the US had pioneered screening of donated blood, the American medical authorities were proclaiming a success. In Britain and France, and many other European countries, the transfusion services were also pleased with the outcome of screening. To the great relief of the British blood transfusion service, the testing seemed to confirm that the initial requests to people whose behaviour put them at high risk to avoid giving blood seemed to have worked. Very few British donors were positive for the virus.

In the US, figures of the number of people who had contracted AIDS from blood transfusions, but who had been infected before screening of blood had begun, showed that the risk was about 1 in 1,000. The percentage of AIDS cases in the US that had occurred as a result of blood transfusions had risen from about 1.2 per cent (12 people) in 1982, to a peak of 2.1 per cent (172 people) in 1985. Children with AIDS had typically caught the virus from contaminated blood. By 1985, the percentage of children with AIDS who had contracted the disease as a result of blood transfusions was over 17 per cent (15 individuals) and rose still further in the following year as more children developed the symptoms as a result of infections that had occurred before the screening began.

The situation in France was not quite so bad. Nevertheless, the screening programme had, for the first time, given a clear indication of how prevalent the virus had become. The first major survey of donated blood, during the second half of 1985, revealed that there were nearly 1,000 HIV-positive batches of blood in nearly 1.5 million donations, which represented about 90 per cent of the country's supply of blood.

This prevalence, approaching 1 in 1,000, worried the French medical authorities. As one scientist who took part in the study said, the measures taken by the French government to persuade people at high risk not to donate blood 'were not fully efficient'.

In Britain, things proved to be a little better. The testing programme had shown that the virus was far less prevalent in those people giving blood in comparison to the US and France. The first big survey, between October 1985 and February 1986, on over a million donors throughout the country, showed that just nineteen were confirmed as being positive for the virus, a prevalence of about 1 in 55,000. In 1987, out of just over 2.5m donations, only twenty-four proved positive for antibodies to HIV. The survey, however, revealed important and startling regional differences. In east Scotland, for instance, which includes the city of Edinburgh, the prevalence of the virus was as high as 1 in about 9,000 donors. A more detailed analysis of high-risk groups showed that about 65 per cent of intravenous drug users in the east of Scotland were antibody positive, whereas just 4.5 per cent of users were positive in the west of Scotland. Clearly there were cultural factors at work, the most likely being that Edinburgh drug users were more likely to share contaminated needles in the back-street 'shooting galleries' of the city than users in west Scotland.

Outside of the developed world, blood testing was far less methodical and frequent. There was another problem, especially in Africa. The tests themselves were more likely to be inaccurate, partly because the reagents in the test could not be stored properly through lack of refrigeration, but also because there are more antibodies in the blood of people in Africa than in people living in more temperate climates. There are more diseases and infections in tropical and semi-tropical areas and so the immune systems of people living there have to cope with a greater variety of foreign micro-organisms entering the body, thus producing more antibodies. Unfortunately, high levels of antibodies in the blood can cause the HIV test to identify an antibody wrongly as one which binds to HIV. Some scientists have described the blood of people living in Africa as 'sticky', meaning that there are many antibodies that can stick to a test kit and so give a false positive. Scientists have reported that the early HIV tests have, for instance, given positive results for people infected with the parasite that causes malaria, although these people are not in fact infected with HIV.

In one study of over 2,500 frozen blood samples that doctors had collected between 1981 and 1984 in five African countries, 9.3 per cent proved positive for HIV overall, and in one country the rate was over 23 per cent. A more detailed analysis of the tests, using the Western blot technique, showed that the vast majority of the positive results were false positives. In this group of people, the scientists could confirm only two blood samples as being antibody positive. The researchers in this study, mainly from the Tropical Diseases Research Centre in Zambia, said that the results they had collected showed that, before 1984, the frequency of HIV in African countries was less than that in many European countries, and that 'the epidemic of AIDS started in central equatorial Africa at about the same time as the epidemic in north America'. A detailed analysis of the results of blood tests in Africa, therefore, seemed to provide little support for the popular notion that the virus had originated there and then spread to the West.

There is one group of people for whom AIDS had become a cruel irony – haemophiliacs. AIDS struck the lives of these people and their families just ten years after improvements in medical technology had at last allowed many haemophiliacs to lead almost normal lives. By the early 1970s, people suffering from even the severest forms of haemophilia could for the first time avoid the once-regular visits to hospital by injecting themselves at home with regular doses of factor VIII, the vital blood-clotting agent collected from blood donors. A decade later, it became apparent that the same batches of life-preserving protein were the cause of an infection with a life-threatening virus.

Long before AIDS was defined, medical scientists knew that treating haemophiliacs with batches of factor VIII made from other people's blood had its risks. The most common problem was, and still is, the contamination of the blood product with the viruses that cause the various types of hepatitis, such as hepatitis-B and non-A-non-B hepatitis, which can lead to severe liver disease, including cancer. The problem with factor VIII is that it is made from up to 30,000 separate donations of blood. In fact, pharmaceuticals companies make factor VIII from blood plasma, the clear liquid in which the red blood cells float. People can donate their blood plasma more frequently than whole blood because it takes longer for the body to replace red blood cells than it does to replace plasma. In the US, people have made money by selling their plasma to pharmaceuticals companies, a trade that many other countries do not permit.

During the manufacture of factor VIII, companies freeze the blood plasma so that the blood proteins, including factor VIII, become concentrated in a 'cryoprecipitate'. Unfortunately, any virus in the pool of plasma also becomes concentrated in the same precipitate. It is very difficult to separate these viruses from the factor VIII. When haemophiliacs began to show the symptoms of AIDS, it confirmed many scientists' early suspicions that a virus was the cause of the problem. The warnings to the community of haemophiliacs, however, came too late for the majority. The virus had already infected many haemophiliacs.

In many countries, such as Britain, France, West Germany and Australia, the proportion of people suffering from severe haemophilia who had become infected with HIV before precautions were taken had risen to well over 50 per cent by 1987. In the US, the proportion approached 100 per cent. Clearly the situation was much worse in the US, and all the evidence suggested that factor VIII imported into European countries from the US was much more likely to be contaminated with HIV than factor VIII made in Europe. One suggestion was that some American companies who paid 'donors' for blood plasma had attracted the wrong clientele because of the financial inducements. The argument was that these donors would be more likely to be people with high-risk behaviour, such as drug users, if they were so poor as to have to sell their plasma. Such people were also less likely to be honest about high-risk activities.

In many countries, including Britain, France and Japan, there was great opposition to importing factor VIII from American sources. In Britain, for instance, the government came under intense pressure to uphold a ten-year-old promise that the country would become self-sufficient in blood products such as factor VIII. In 1987, however, the promise had still not been fulfilled. According to the Haemophilia Society, a British charity representing 5,000 haemophiliacs, Britain was making only a fifth of the nation's total demand for factor VIII in 1987: 'If the UK had processed sufficient voluntary donated plasma into factor VIII,' the society said, 'the number of people infected would be substantially less because the use of heavily contaminated material from abroad would have been avoided.'

In 1984, scientists discovered that heating factor VIII to high enough temperatures could kill certain viruses, such as hepatitis viruses, the same way that pasteurizing milk kills many of the bacteria in milk. By 1985, most companies and laboratories making factor VIII had begun to heat it during the manufacturing process to kill HIV. A year later, however, some doctors treating haemophiliacs began to have suspicions about whether heat treatment actually worked. A handful of haemophiliacs had apparently developed antibodies to HIV a year after being given the heat-treated factor VIII. The question was whether they had become infected with virus that had survived the treatment or whether they had taken more than a year to seroconvert.

The company at the centre of the controversy, Armour Pharmaceuticals of the US, decided to recall certain batches of its product from the market. The British government later withdrew Armour's licence to sell factor VIII in the UK because of the fears associated with its product. Armour's manufacturing process involved heating factor VIII to 60°C for 30 minutes. The Blood Products Laboratory, a government establishment at Elstree in Hertfordshire, recommended that factor VIII should be heated to 60°C for 72 hours. The disadvantage of higher temperatures for longer periods, however, is that more factor VIII is destroyed in the process and so the product becomes more expensive to make, although safer.

Armour decided to develop a method of cleaning up factor VIII that would produce a much purer product, free of virus. The method, developed by researchers in California in the early 1980s, was to filter the factor VIII through a column of antibodies. These would behave like tiny magnets pulling out molecules of factor VIII and letting anything else pass through. In this way, the company believed, the final product would be more than 99 per cent pure, and would not even need to be heat treated, although this could be done for extra safety. The company received a licence to sell the product in the US in 1987.

The ultimate breakthrough for haemophiliacs, however, will be the manufacture of factor VIII by the new science of genetic engineering. The idea is to insert a gene that can make factor VIII into a microorganism, which, when grown in bulk, will then produce the human blood protein in large quantities for harvesting. There is even one plan to insert the human factor VIII gene into cows so that the protein can be collected in the animals' milk.

Genetically engineered factor VIII and heat-treated factor VIII have come too late for the thousands of haemophiliacs throughout the world who have become infected with contaminated blood products. Many hundreds of them have already developed AIDS, and some have died. Dozens of wives and lovers of haemophiliac men have learnt that they, too, have become infected with the virus. They, like their antibody-positive partners, live in the knowledge that AIDS is a real possibility. The development of a blood test has been a blessing to many who would have otherwise received contaminated blood products or blood transfusions, and who would have possibly infected their sexual partners as well. To many others, however, the test has brought only the frightening prospect of premature death.

Chapter 7

ANATOMY OF A VIRUS

It is a bizarre fact of life that an organism as simple as a virus can cause a disease as dreaded and deadly as AIDS. Once scientists had identified the human immunodeficiency virus, the race was on to find drugs that would conquer it, or a vaccine that would prevent its spread. But first researchers had to find out every intimate detail they could about it. Their efforts have been unprecedented. Never in the history of medicine have scientists found out so much about a disease in such a short time. By the late 1980s, they probably knew more about the human immunodeficiency virus than about any other virus.

One of the most fundamental characteristics of HIV is the unusual way in which it stores its genetic information. This is in the form of ribonucleic acid (RNA). Most living organisms, by contrast, have genetic material in the form of deoxyribonucleic acid (DNA). The DNA is the blueprint of life: it carries the genetic information unique to the organism. This information is held in the form of the particular sequence of the small molecules that make up the long strand of DNA – equivalent, in the analogy used on p. 44, to the beads of a necklace. From this sequence of molecules, the cells of plants and animals make a mirror-image or complementary version of the genetic material. This copy is called RNA. The RNA contains the information that the cell needs in order to make proteins.

Proteins are vital components of living organisms. These molecules are made up of strings of smaller molecules, called amino acids. These strings are often folded, giving the protein a specific shape which reflects the molecule's function. Proteins come in a huge variety. Some are structural and highly specialized, such as those that make up human hair and nails. Other proteins may be involved in the daily life of a cell, making sure that it responds to signals, or receives enough food and oxygen, or eliminates waste materials. Some of these proteins will be of a type called enzymes. Enzymes play an important role in carrying out certain chemical reactions in the body. Enzymes in the human gut, for example, break down food into a form that the body can absorb.

Most living organisms manufacture their own proteins. Viruses, in contrast, have to hijack the cellular machinery of other organisms in order to make proteins. A virus is not a complete cell: it has only some genetic material and a protective 'coat' of protein. It is not alive in the strict sense of the word, for it has no means of reproducing itself – until it enters a cell of its host.

Some viruses contain DNA as their genetic material. Once the virus has attached itself to the host cell and inserted its DNA, the cell is deceived into making viral proteins. Some of these proteins are the enzymes necessary for the synthesis of more viral DNA. Many new viruses assemble themselves from these component parts, bursting free from the host cell, which may die in the process.

Other viruses, including HIV, contain RNA instead of DNA. As explained earlier, HIV belongs to a family of viruses named the retroviruses. 'Retro' means backwards, and retroviruses are so called because the virus persuades the host cell to convert viral RNA back into DNA, contrary to the cell's normal method of operation, which involves making RNA from DNA. When HIV infects a cell, its outer envelope fuses with the membrane of the cell (see figure 6). This releases viral RNA into the cell, along with an enzyme which tells the

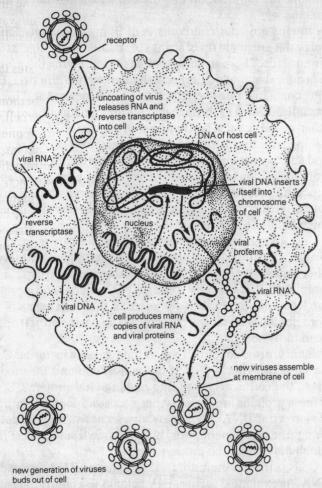

HIV

receptor

uncoating of virus
releases RNA and
reverse transcriptase
into cell

viral RNA

reverse
transcriptase

DNA of host cell

viral DNA inserts
itself into
chromosome
of cell

nucleus

viral
proteins

viral RNA

viral DNA

cell produces many
copies of viral RNA
and viral proteins

new viruses assemble
at membrane of cell

new generation of viruses
buds out of cell

Figure 6. The life cycle of the human immunodeficiency virus. It takes over the cell's machinery for making proteins, channelling the activity of the cell into the manufacture of many new viruses.

cell to make DNA from the RNA. This enzyme, as we said in Chapter 3, is called reverse transcriptase. It is unique to retroviruses and does not occur in human cells. Such individuality may be important when it comes to designing drugs to combat HIV infection, for the trick is to find some way of knocking out the virus without destroying the human cells in which it lives.

The viral DNA then enters the nucleus and integrates itself into the DNA of the cell. Once there, the viral DNA lies dormant. This is the latent stage of infection. It can last for months or years. Eventually, when some trigger activates the cell, the viral DNA starts to direct the production of viral components. There are many theories about what the trigger might be. For example, there is some evidence that subsequent infections with other viruses, such as herpes viruses, can activate infected cells. Whatever the trigger, the result is the manufacture of viral protein and viral RNA – the two main components of HIV. The viral proteins migrate to the surface of the host cell, where they stick out through its outer membrane. The remaining elements of the virus, including the RNA, also assemble themselves beneath the cell membrane. Then, by a process known as budding, multitudes of new viruses detach themselves from the host cell, borne away in the bloodstream to attack other cells. Each virus has a diameter of only 0.1 micrometres. A cube containing a thousand million viruses would measure just one tenth of a millimetre across – barely visible to the naked eye.

During budding, the virus takes part of the cell's outer fatty membrane with it. Molecules of protein sit at regular intervals in this viral membrane or envelope (see figure 7). These proteins are called glycoproteins because they have molecules of sugar attached to them. HIV has two glycoproteins, called gp120 and gp41. The 'gp' stands for glycoprotein; the numbers reflect the sizes of the molecules. The viral membrane also bears proteins called HLA, or 'cellular' antigens, which are derived from the membrane of the host cell.

Inside the viral envelope is a structure called the core shell. This layer may be made of a protein known as p18. Some researchers believe that the core shell has a faceted appearance. The core shell conceals the core itself, which contains the genetic material of HIV, the RNA. The core,

97

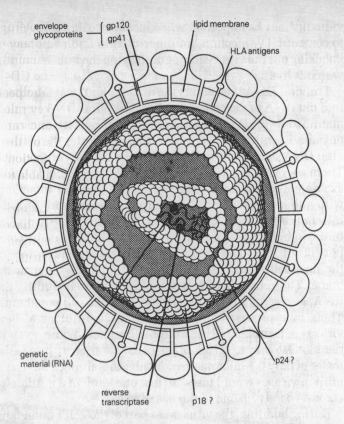

envelope glycoproteins { gp120 gp41

lipid membrane

HLA antigens

genetic material (RNA)

reverse transcriptase

p18 ?

p24 ?

Figure 7. A model of the structure of the virus. The virus derives its lipid membrane from the human cell by a process of budding.

which may be made of a protein called p24, seems to have a highly organized structure too, being in the form of a hollow cone. Studies with powerful electron microscopes suggest that the narrow end of this cone is open, while the wider, closed end is dimpled, rather like the base of a champagne bottle. Scientists believe that the enzyme reverse transcriptase, so vital to the virus's success in attacking cells, is associated with the RNA in the core of the virus.

The virus attacks human cells with the help of the glycoproteins in its envelope. These carry a special binding site that recognizes and attaches to another type of glycoprotein, a molecule called CD4, which is found on the membranes of some human cells, particularly some cells of the immune system. One of the commonest kinds of cell to carry the CD4 molecule is the type of white blood cell called the T-helper cell. Other cells, called macrophages, which play a key role in eliminating invading microbes, also carry CD4 and can become infected with HIV. This affinity to cells of the immune system is the key to the paradox of HIV infection. HIV attacks the very cells which should normally be able to help to eliminate it.

The function of a person's immune system is to recognize and eliminate foreign substances, called antigens, that have entered the body. Any foreign material can act as an antigen, whether it is the protein coat of a bacterium or a virus, a cancer cell, or a transplanted organ. Every individual encounters scores of antigens every day. Most of the time, the cells and molecules that police the body for antigens deal with the intruder. At other times, perhaps because the body has never encountered that antigen before, the person succumbs to the infection. Eventually the body mounts an immune response and usually manages to fight off the bacterium or virus concerned. A key element in this response is the production of antibodies, protein molecules that recognize and bind to specific antigens and help to eliminate them.

Complex interactions between many types of cells and molecules – not just antibodies – regulate the immune response. Some of the cells have the task of engulfing foreign particles. Macrophages, for example, are large cells that can swallow and destroy bacteria and, sometimes, viruses. Other cells that take a key part in the immune response are the lymphocytes – white blood cells. There are two types of lymphocyte, T-cells and B-cells. When a B-cell encounters an antigen that it recognizes, it becomes transformed into a plasma cell (see figure 8). Plasma cells manufacture quantities of antibodies that recognize the original antigen. The antibodies bind to the antigen, inactivating it in a variety of ways. Antibodies that

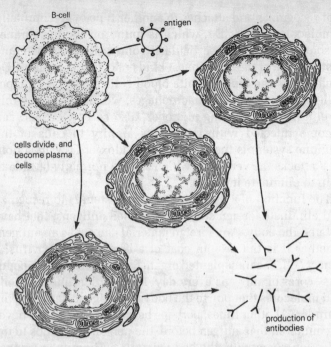

B-cell

antigen

cells divide and
become plasma
cells

production of
antibodies

Figure 8. Antigens stimulate B-cells to divide and mature into specialized cells called plasma cells. These cells manufacture antibodies that recognize the original antigen. In people with AIDS, some B-cells produce antibodies at the wrong times while others fail to respond to new antibodies when they should.

bind to bacteria, for example, may make it easier for macrophages to engulf and kill these microorganisms.

Viruses, unlike bacteria, are not alive in the strict sense of the word because they have no means of reproducing until they invade a host cell. So scientists talk about neutralizing viruses, rather than killing them. In many cases, antibodies can neutralize viruses, perhaps by binding to the virus at the point where the virus normally attacks the cell. The body can then eliminate the virus. Antibodies that are capable of this feat are called 'neutralizing antibodies'. Unfortunately for people infected with HIV, the body produces only low levels

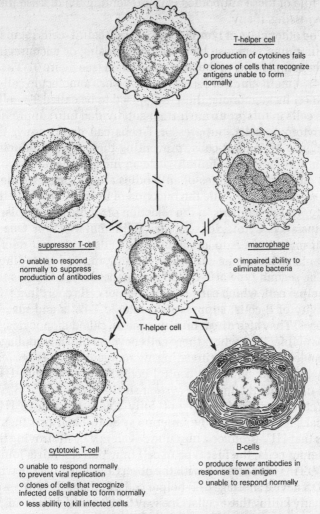

T-helper cell
o production of cytokines fails
o clones of cells that recognize antigens unable to form normally

suppressor T-cell
o unable to respond normally to suppress production of antibodies

macrophage
o impaired ability to eliminate bacteria

T-helper cell

cytotoxic T-cell
o unable to respond normally to prevent viral replication
o clones of cells that recognize infected cells unable to form normally
o less ability to kill infected cells

B-cells
o produce fewer antibodies in response to an antigen
o unable to respond normally

Figure 9. The T-cell plays a central role in the immune system.

of neutralizing antibodies against this virus, and they seem to be unable to eliminate the infection. By the late 1980s, scientists had still not discovered why this is so, or what the role of these antibodies is in preventing the disease from progressing, if any.

The other class of lymphocyte is the T-cell. T-cells regulate the immune response by either suppressing or encouraging other components of the immune system (see figure 9). There are two main kinds of T-cell. One type has a molecule called CD8 on its membrane; these cells used to be called T8-cells. The cells in this group are further subdivided into suppressor or cytotoxic cells. Suppressor T-cells can damp down the response of some B-cells, preventing them from producing their antibodies indefinitely once an infection is under control and such quantities of antibodies are no longer needed. These cells also initiate the rejection of foreign cells from the body, which happens in the rejection of an organ transplant, for instance. Cytotoxic cells have a different function. One of their main tasks is to attack infected cells to prevent microorganisms inside the cells from multiplying and spreading.

The second type of T-cell, the type that HIV infects, is the T-helper cell, which carries CD4. Helper cells coordinate the activity of B-cells, suppressor-cytotoxic T-cells and macrophages. They also direct immature cells, called monocytes, to sites of infection, where these cells develop into macrophages capable of eliminating invading microorganisms. It is because T-helper cells have this central coordinating role that HIV can devastate the immune system so effectively.

Yet immunologists do not fully understand how HIV wreaks its damage on the immune system. Their first theory was that HIV produced immune deficiency by destroying the T-helper cells, the first type of cell in which scientists found HIV. This idea fitted in with the observation that people with AIDS have a shortage of T-helper cells. Perhaps the virus was directly killing these cells. One way that it could do this might be by replicating and producing many progeny viruses, so that the cell bursts and dies. An alternative theory depended on the fact that infected cells carry on their membranes not only CD4 receptors – the proteins that HIV recognizes – but also viral envelope proteins that have migrated to the membrane in preparation for the budding of new viruses. The CD4

102

receptors on uninfected T-cells will bind to the viral proteins on the surfaces of infected cells. So if two infected cells meet, or an infected cell comes into contact with an uninfected T-helper cell, the two cells can bind together. Adjacent parts of the membrane of an infected cell could also become bound to each other, disrupting the normal configuration and activity of the cell.

Scientists frequently observe this kind of interaction when they grow batches of infected cells in the laboratory. The result is that many cells merge, forming large structures with many nuclei, called syncytia, which do not survive for long. But it is not always possible to establish what happens in the body from laboratory observations such as these. Although some researchers have seen large cells with many nuclei in some tissues from patients with AIDS, particularly from the brain, this seems to be quite rare. Many scientists believe that, if this mechanism were the main cause for the dearth of T-helper cells, they would have found it much more often in patients.

The other problem with this theory is that, in patients, relatively few T-helper cells seem to be infected with the virus. Only about one in 10,000 to one in 100,000 lymphocytes in the circulating blood are actively infected with the virus (although rather more may contain DNA derived from the virus). Even if all these infected cells were to die, however, the rate at which the body replaces its T-helper lymphocytes ought to be enough to compensate for this loss.

Of course, the mechanism for replacing T-cells could be at fault. One theory is that HIV may infect and kill the cells in the bone marrow which, when they mature, give rise to T-helper lymphocytes. By killing one of these cells, which are called stem cells, HIV could in one stroke remove that cell's capability to produce a multitude of mature T-helper lymphocytes.

Another possibility is that the body's own cytotoxic cells turn on T-helper cells infected with HIV and destroy them. Infected T-cells frequently display viral proteins on their surface. Cytotoxic T-cells might then recognize the infected cells as foreign and kill them.

Some effect of the virus on *uninfected* T-helper cells may be to blame. Perhaps viral envelope protein, because it binds to the CD4 receptor, somehow blocks the function that this receptor normally performs. In 1988, however, researchers in the US put forward another theory. Results of their experiments suggested a mechanism by which uninfected T-helper cells could become the victims of the body's cytotoxic T-cells. These experiments were carried out only in the laboratory: scientists have yet to prove their relevance to what goes on in the body. But the work has provided new insights into how cells of the immune system deal with the virus.

The theory is as follows. Scientists know that the envelope protein of the virus, gp120, tends to come off the intact virus very easily. So gp120 is likely to be present in the blood of infected people in whom the virus is actively replicating. When a foreign antigen (such as a microorganism, or, in this case, the viral protein) comes into contact with cells of the immune system, it will normally be engulfed by cells such as macrophages. Inside the macrophage, the antigen is broken down into fragments which then migrate to the surface of the cell. The cell then 'presents' the foreign proteins to other cells, such as T-cells, in order to activate them. This may result, for example, in the T-cell releasing substances which disrupt the membrane of the macrophage. This process, called lysis, spells the end for any microorganism infecting the macrophage.

Only specialized cells such as macrophages can normally present antigens in this way to other cells of the immune system. Normally, T-cells cannot present antigens because they have no way of taking up antigens. But gp120 is different, as the researchers showed. Because this viral protein can bind directly to the cell, the cell can take it in, break it down and display the fragments on the cell membrane. Other T-cells in the body can then kill the antigen-presenting T-cell.

The researchers called these assassins 'cytolytic' cells (literally, cells capable of lysis). In people never exposed to HIV, cytolytic T-cells that recognize gp120 are very rare. Nevertheless, the researchers managed to identify some, and show that these cells could indeed kill T-helper cells that had been exposed to gp120. The cruel twist to this theory is that the cytolytic cells are capable of killing these T-helper cells only if they have a second type of protein displayed on their surfaces. This protein is normally found on some human cells, but it appears on the surface of T-helper cells only when these are activated to fight an infection. So, only *activated* T-helper cells exposed to viral gp120 would be vulnerable to destruction by cytolytic cells primed to recognize the viral protein. And someone who loses activated T-cells can no longer fight certain infections.

Loss of T-helper cells is not the only abnormality in the immune systems of people infected with HIV. Those T-helper cells that remain do not function normally. For example, some researchers have shown that T-helper cells from HIV-infected people do not respond normally to a stimulus from an antigen that would usually cause them to divide and proliferate. T-cells stimulated in this way also normally produce a chemical signal called interleukin-2. This chemical stimulates other T-cells to grow and mature. T-cells that are infected with HIV, however, produce abnormally low amounts of interleukin-2 when stimulated.

The T-helper cell is not the only cell of the immune system that HIV infects. Macrophages, and their immature forms, monocytes, are also susceptible to the virus. They may become infected when they engulf the virus. These cells also have CD4 molecules on their surfaces, to which HIV can attach, though these molecules are more sparsely distributed on macrophages than on the membranes of T-helper cells. The virus seems to affect macrophages differently. Infected macrophages, instead of producing viral particles on their surfaces, accumulate them inside the cell. Macrophages grown in the laboratory can be full of viruses, and yet survive. They may even be capable of 'secreting' viruses. It also seems probable that these cells are responsible for carrying the virus around the body, particularly to the brain.

Infection of monocytes and macrophages, which have an important role in presenting antigens to T-helper cells in order to activate them, may account for some of the defects in the immune system in AIDS. Alternatively, the abnormalities observed in macrophages isolated from people with AIDS may occur because T-helper cells do not stimulate them normally. As with T-helper cells, however, only a small proportion of monocytes in the circulating blood are infected.

Researchers have also shown in laboratory experiments that it is possible to infect some of the immature cells of the bone marrow with HIV. These cells – known as 'stem cells' – were of a group which develops into monocytes and macrophages. This raises the possibility that macrophages become infected very early on in their life cycle, while the stem cells are still in the bone marrow. Infected cells in the bone marrow could also pass on the virus to lymphocytes passing through the marrow. The researchers next planned to find out whether their observations in the laboratory also held true in patients.

Surprisingly, the stem cells which became infected displayed no detectable molecules of CD4, the receptor which scientists formerly believed was essential for the virus to lock on to the cell. Many researchers still believe that CD4 must be present for HIV infection to occur: they maintain that if a cell has the genetic message for CD4, even if it is not making that protein in quantities large enough for scientists to detect, HIV will still be able to infect the cell. Only one molecule of CD4 needs to be present for the virus to get in, they point out. HIV infection may be the most sensitive test available for whether CD4 is present.

On the other hand, there has been an increasing number of reports of HIV infecting other cells – some types of brain cell, for example – which appear to have no CD4. Adding antibodies that normally block the interaction between the virus and CD4 were unable to prevent HIV infecting these types of cells. This is worrying for researchers, because it could mean that many of the strategies for drugs and vaccines, which depend on blocking the interaction between the virus and the CD4 receptor on the T-cell, may not work. By late

106

1988, however, there was no firm answer to the question of whether the virus could enter cells without interacting in some way with CD4.

The complex and unusual biology of HIV has led some scientists to question even whether the virus is the true cause of AIDS. The most articulate proponent of this heresy is Peter Duesberg, a professor of molecular biology at the University of California, Berkeley. Duesberg made his ideas known in a paper published in March 1987 in the journal *Cancer Research*. For a year following the publication of his rather esoteric theory, the scientific establishment all but ignored the points he raised. The result was that some sections of the popular press began to look upon the maverick Duesberg as a *cause célèbre*.

Articles in *Spin*, a rock music paper that was one of the first to interview Duesberg, and *New York Native*, a gay newspaper, brought Duesberg's ideas to a wider, less scientifically literate, audience. His arguments were extremely powerful and seductive. Many people began to believe that Duesberg could be right and that the silence from the scientific establishment was only confirmation that leading AIDS researchers had made a dreadful mistake – HIV may not, after all, be the cause of AIDS. In Britain, a television documentary, called *The Unheard Voices*, fuelled the Duesberg controversy, and won an award in so doing. The silence from the ivory towers of the scientific establishment, meanwhile, was deafening.

Duesberg had even said that he would be prepared to have himself injected with pure HIV to prove that it was a harmless passenger in people with AIDS. He had not, however, carried out his threat because pure HIV was virtually impossible to guarantee. Nevertheless, Duesberg's arguments grew in stature, and the 'AIDS establishment' had finally to answer the questions that he had raised.

His convoluted arguments rested on several points. Central to these was his assertion that HIV fails to conform to Koch's postulates, named after the great German bacteriologist

107

Robert Koch, who won a Nobel prize in 1905 for his work on human diseases. The postulates state that for a microorganism to cause a disease, it must follow certain rules. The organism must be present in all cases of the disease, scientists must be able to cultivate it separately from any other microorganisms, reinoculation of the microbe into a susceptible animal must reproduce the disease, and scientists must be able to reisolate the microorganism from the infected animal and cultivate it again in pure culture.

It must be said that Koch's postulates are rarely, if ever, fulfilled. They are largely theoretical, rather than practical. There are, for instance, many cases of tuberculosis where it is difficult to isolate and culture the causative agent, *Mycobacterium tuberculosis*, from infected individuals. As one British scientist, Jonathan Weber of the Royal Postgraduate Medical School in London, remarked: 'If Koch himself had been required to culture *M. tuberculosis* from every clinical case of TB he saw, his postulates would have been stillborn.'

Duesberg argued that it is not possible to detect HIV in every person suffering from AIDS, and that HIV does not cause AIDS when it is injected into chimpanzees, or accidentally into healthy humans. AIDS researchers say, however, that it may have been true that in the early years scientists found it difficult to find HIV in all cases of AIDS. But new techniques for detecting HIV, they say, have shown that it is now possible to find HIV 'in essentially all AIDS patients'. It is indeed true that HIV does not so far appear to cause AIDS in chimps, but there are many viruses that cause disease in humans but fail to cause illness in animals. Duesberg's other statement – that HIV does not cause AIDS in people accidentally inoculated with it – is categorically denied by AIDS researchers. About one in every 100 nurses and health workers who have accidentally pricked themselves with needles contaminated with blood infected with HIV have developed antibodies to HIV, and some have developed AIDS.

Duesberg had many other arguments in support of his contention that HIV is but a harmless passenger in AIDS patients. 'It is paradoxical,' he said, that HIV is said to cause AIDS on the grounds that people at risk of it have developed antibodies to the virus. 'Viruses typically cause disease only in the absence of antibodies to the virus, which neutralize the virulence of the virus. This is why vaccination works so well,' he said. 'This is all the more paradoxical because this virus does not become activated when the carrier of the virus develops the symptoms of AIDS. Thus HIV is the only virus that seems to cause disease after rather than before the development of antibodies.'

This argument ignores that fact that it is common for viruses to stimulate the production of antibodies which do not protect against the effects of that virus. In people infected with herpes, for instance, the virus can often become active some time after doctors find high levels of antibodies in the blood that are specific to that virus. The same goes for other common infections, such as measles, where people can suffer from late complications even in the presence of high levels of antibodies to the microbe.

Duesberg came up with several more arguments in support of his contention. HIV, he said, is not biochemically active in people with AIDS. It only infects a minute proportion of T-cells, a level of infection that the body could easily withstand. 'Under these conditions,' he said, 'HIV cannot account for the loss of T-cells, the hallmark of AIDS, even if all infected cells died. This is because during the two days it takes for HIV to replicate, the body regenerates about 5 per cent of its T-cells, more than enough to compensate for losses due to HIV.'

This was a difficult point for AIDS researchers to answer. They had little idea how HIV causes depletion of T-cells *in vivo* – though they had lots of ideas from experiments *in vitro*. Nevertheless, they said that Duesberg conveniently ignored the fact that HIV also infects the stem cells, the cells that divide and proliferate to produce mature blood cells. Obviously, if the stem cells are being depleted, then the effects on the numbers of cells in the blood will be profound.

Yet another point that Duesberg raised was that HIV seems

109

to behave differently according to whom it infects, and where. 'No known virus or microbe discriminates between men and women, nor between homosexuals and heterosexuals,' he said. AIDS affects predominantly homosexual men in the West, yet it affects both men and women in equal proportions in Africa. The virus is said to cause Kaposi's sarcoma in homosexuals in the US, yet diarrhoea, weight loss and fever are the main symptoms in people in Africa, he said. How can one virus cause different symptoms?

The answer is that environmental and genetic factors could both influence the way the disease progresses in a person infected with HIV. Furthermore, AIDS researchers argue that the distribution of HIV mirrors the distribution of AIDS in the world, an association that shows that HIV causes AIDS. It is also common for infectious agents to affect certain groups differently. Hepatitis-B virus, which is also spread sexually, affects predominantly homosexual men in the West. Syphilis affects fourteen men to every woman in Britain – whereas the proportion was 50:50 several decades ago when syphilis was still rampant in the heterosexual community. Nowadays, most cases in Britain are among homosexuals.

Duesberg practically ignored the most important reason for believing that HIV causes AIDS: there is a welter of data showing that where one finds HIV, one also finds AIDS. It is true for a retrospective analysis of how the disease succeeded in reaching haemophiliacs and people who received blood transfusions. And it is true for an analysis of those who have AIDS today, and those who are infected with HIV. A reply to Duesberg by several AIDS scientists, published in Science in 1988, states: 'Numerous studies have shown that in countries with no persons with HIV antibodies there is no AIDS, and in countries with many persons with HIV antibodies there is much AIDS.'

In those children infected with HIV from their mothers, 95 per cent develop AIDS within six years, whereas their uninfected siblings never develop AIDS. In twin babies where one received a contaminated blood transfusion, that infant developed AIDS whereas the other twin and the

110

mother did not. 'Blocking the transmission of HIV prevents the occurrence of AIDS,' scientists said. The cause is HIV; the effect is AIDS.

For many scientists, Duesberg is an irrelevant distraction. For others, he is a dangerous apologist for those who want to believe that those infected with HIV or at risk of infection with HIV can carry on with 'business as usual'. But for some people, perhaps those most in need of the explanations, Duesberg has served a useful function in raising important questions about HIV that needed answering outside the rarefied atmosphere of virology. Without Duesberg, perhaps no one would have bothered to justify why HIV, a virus with such an extraordinary biology, is the cause of the immune suppression that results in AIDS.

Chapter 8

IN THE GRIP OF THE VIRUS

Whatever the exact causes of the failure of the immune system in people with AIDS, the effect seems to be largely the same. Most people infected with the virus develop severe immuno-deficiency. They are no longer able to fight off infections and malignant cells. Various viruses, bacteria and other micro-organisms seize their opportunity and multiply while the body's defences are down. The defects in immunity also allow certain cancers to develop. People with AIDS are prone to a type of skin cancer called Kaposi's sarcoma, and to another kind of cancer called lymphoma, which develops in the lymph glands.

In the few years since doctors first described the syndrome of infections and tumours known as AIDS, researchers have been hard at work untangling the new evidence about the course of the disease. During the late 1980s, medical scientists established a great deal about how the body responds to infec-tion with HIV. Much of this information has become avail-able as a result of the development of new tests.

As already mentioned, the first tests capable of telling whether someone was infected with HIV relied on the detec-tion of antibodies. By 1988, however, the polymerase chain reaction test (described on p. 79) had become available. This test makes it possible to detect the presence of viral genetic material even if a sample contains only minute traces of the virus. One surprising observation made possible by this test is that antibodies to the virus can take months and even years to develop.

The first indication that such a delay might occur came from research published in 1987 by Finnish and American scientists. They studied twenty-five men who were the sexual partners of infected men. The twenty-five were not infected, according to the standard screening test for antibodies, the ELISA test. When the researchers used alternative tests available at that time to look for other signs of the virus, such as viral antigen and viral genetic material, they found evidence of infection in five of the men long before the ELISA test detected antibodies. These signs were present between sixteen and thirty-four months earlier. In stored samples of serum from another nine people diagnosed as infected with HIV, viral proteins and viral genetic material appeared as much as six to fourteen months before an ELISA test could detect antibodies.

The polymerase chain reaction (PCR) test has shed further light on the early stages of infection. American researchers announced at the Fourth International Conference on AIDS, in June 1988, that PCR could detect signs of the virus in some people at high risk of infection up to forty-two months earlier than conventional tests could. The researchers studied blood samples taken from forty-one homosexual and bisexual men living in four American cities. Between April 1984 and March 1985, eighteen men in the group developed antibodies to HIV (in other words, they seroconverted). The scientists used PCR to study the blood samples taken from these men before they seroconverted. They found signs of HIV in sixteen of the men at least six months before these people developed antibodies that could be detected by the most sensitive antibody test – the Western blot test. In four men, PCR revealed that HIV was present two years before seroconversion. One man had been infected with HIV for at least thirty-six months before seroconversion and another for forty-two months.

The evidence from PCR raises the worrying possibility that some people may have been falsely reassured on the basis of an antibody test that they were not infected. Anthony Fauci, director of the National Institute of Allergy and Infectious Diseases in the US, has said that people who have been at very high risk of HIV infection, such as the regular sexual partners of infected people, yet have had negative tests for antibodies should be aware of the possibility that they could be infected. They may want to be tested again by PCR. (Provided technical difficulties have been overcome, this could be more generally available by 1989/90.) Fauci said that there was no way of knowing how many people were seronegative but nevertheless infected. But it was unlikely that 'millions of people' were infected who had previously thought they were in the clear, he added.

How does this evidence fit in with what scientists know about the life cycle of the virus? One theory is that HIV has two options when it enters the body. It can either integrate its DNA into the cells it has infected, without replicating and releasing virus into the blood. In this case, which Fauci has called latent infection, no antibodies would be produced. Possibly, the virus is just sitting quietly in the body's macrophages during this stage. There it would remain until some trigger sets off viral replication. Alternatively, the virus might begin actively replicating as soon as it enters the body.

Scientists are not sure what determines whether the virus remains latent. Perhaps the route of infection plays a role, or the form in which the recipient's cells first encounter the virus: the virus may enter the body inside infected cells, or it may be floating free in the bloodstream.

To find free virus in the blood, researchers take a sample of blood from a seropositive person and remove the blood cells. They then look for viruses in the fluid that remains. Such studies have shown that it is possible to find free virus in about one in every three such samples from seropositive people. There are usually about ten viruses, or 'infectious particles', as researchers call them, per millilitre. (A standard teaspoon holds 5 millilitres.) Levels of virus in semen and vaginal fluids are even lower. However, infected cells are

114

often present in great quantities in semen (especially in men with sexually transmitted diseases and related infections).

Some researchers have therefore suggested that infected white blood cells may play an important role in the sexual transmission of HIV. In homosexual men, for example, the infected cells could enter the body of the receptive partner either through small tears in the skin of the anal canal, or by coming into contact with, and directly infecting, susceptible cells in the lining of the bowel. Similar mechanisms could account for transmission from men to women and women to men via vaginal intercourse, although the risk of infection from each route is likely to vary. (Direct transfer of free virus could still occur, of course, if virus in semen or vaginal fluids entered the bloodstream through abrasions of the skin.)

Some researchers have put forward the theory that a very long latency period before seroconversion may result if the virus enters the body inside infected cells. Conversely, if free virus enters the bloodstream directly, as might occur in intravenous drug users, the course of the infection might be more rapid.

Progress in determining whether this theory holds true will be slow, however, because studies to determine the period between infection and the production of antibodies are so difficult to carry out. Many people do not know exactly when they were exposed to the virus. Investigations carried out on the handful of health-care workers who have become infected after stabbing themselves with a needle contaminated with blood from infected patients have shown that antibodies generally appear a few weeks to a few months after exposure to the virus. But the discoveries made possible by the polymerase chain reaction test suggest that antibodies may take much longer to appear following sexual transmission of the virus, in some cases at least.

The polymerase chain reaction test seems to be raising as many questions as it answers. Another strange observation is that people who have developed antibodies to HIV may, in rare cases, subsequently lose them. American researchers reported in 1988 that four homosexual men, who had anti-

115

bodies to the virus when initially tested, were later negative for antibodies, even on the sensitive Western blot test. The PCR test allowed the scientists to show that the genetic material of HIV was still present in the men's blood. None of these men was ill, and all had normal levels of T-helper cells. The researchers suggested that the virus may have failed to replicate sufficiently in these men to trigger sustained production of antibodies at levels high enough for tests to detect.

One further unexpected finding was that later PCR tests on the blood of two of the men were negative. The scientists say that these men may still be infected with HIV, but the virus may be in a latent state somewhere in the body, such as the brain, where a PCR test on the person's blood cannot detect it. Loss of antibodies does not seem to suggest that the body has conquered the virus, the researchers warn. They plan to carry on studying these men, to find out whether the infection becomes active again and the antibodies reappear.

Some of the scientists who first discovered that antibodies could take more than a year to appear have also tried to determine what factors stimulated the development of antibodies in people with latent infection. They found that a full antibody response occurred only after the individuals had become infected with other viruses such as cytomegalovirus, Epstein-Barr virus (which causes glandular fever, also known as mononucleosis) or hepatitis-B virus. These viruses all contain DNA, and the researchers suggested that they might play a role in enhancing the replication of HIV.

Whatever determines the length of the latent period before antibodies develop, many people report having a minor illness shortly after their first exposure to the virus, just before antibodies appear. This illness is similar to many other viral diseases, such as influenza, glandular fever or rubella (German measles). Those individuals affected feel tired and unwell, with aching muscles and joints. They may have a sore throat, swollen lymph glands, a high temperature, a headache, a rash or diarrhoea. Symptoms that indicate that the nervous system is involved may appear: the person may become confused and disorientated, with loss of memory or changes in personality. These symptoms last for about eight to twelve days, and the person usually recovers without the need for medical attention.

Tests carried out at this time show that viral antigens, particularly the core protein called p24, are present in the blood. Yet tests for antibodies usually prove negative at this stage. Although there are exceptions (as described above) in most people, antibodies take two weeks to three months to appear following infection. At around the time that the antibodies develop, the core protein of the virus, the p24 antigen, vanishes. This disappearance may be the result of a temporary immune response. A period of silent infection then begins, during which most people remain well. This period can last for months or years. Yet a proportion of people will at some point experience symptoms caused by the infection.

There are several patterns of illness caused by infection with HIV, some of which are eventually classified as AIDS if the symptoms become severe enough. Many people infected with the virus develop persistently enlarged lymph nodes. This condition is called persistent generalized lymphadenopathy (PGL) or lymphadenopathy syndrome (LAS). In many cases, the development of PGL is what prompts the person to visit a doctor. The enlarged lymph nodes appear most commonly in the neck and the armpit and under the jaw. (Enlarged nodes in the groin do not count in the definition of this syndrome, because such swelling commonly occurs as a result of other sexually transmitted infections.) The affected nodes are symmetrical – for example, in both armpits – and at least one centimetre in diameter. They do not feel tender.

Some people progress to PGL early on in the course of infection while in others this is a late development. Doctors have carried out many studies to try to determine the significance of PGL and whether this condition makes it more or less likely that the person concerned will develop AIDS. So far, research suggests that the risk of someone with persistently swollen lymph glands developing AIDS during a five-year period is between 10 and 30 per cent – about the same as for all HIV-infected people. Other studies have found no

117

correlation between the severity of lymphadenopathy and the degree of damage to the immune system.

Some people with persistently swollen lymph glands are otherwise healthy. Others experience a range of symptoms of varying severity. People infected with the virus but without swollen lymph glands may also develop these symptoms. These conditions include fatigue, diarrhoea, night sweats, weight loss of over 10 per cent, and persistent fever. The symptoms may persist or may appear intermittently, lasting for several weeks at a time.

Before the advent of the test for antibodies to HIV, doctors used to use the term AIDS-related complex (ARC) to describe these types of symptoms. Someone had ARC if they had two or more such symptoms for three months or longer, together with two or more abnormal laboratory tests, such as low levels of T-helper cells. But the term ARC is less commonly used now that the definition of AIDS itself has changed. The new definition, formulated by the Centers for Disease Control in Atlanta, came into effect in September 1987. It included for the first time the group of symptoms known as 'HIV wasting syndrome' or, in Africa, 'slim disease'. These symptoms include severe loss of weight and diarrhoea, which may be accompanied by fever. Patients with this syndrome, formerly classified as having ARC, are now said to have AIDS.

Other problems that people infected with HIV may experience include skin rashes and viral and fungal infections. These include tinea (ringworm), thrush (a fungal infection) affecting the mouth, herpes simplex (oral or genital) and herpes zoster (shingles). Attacks of herpes are more severe and last longer than in healthy people. Tooth decay, mouth ulcers and dental abscesses may also occur. One condition, formerly very rare, which occurs in people infected with HIV, is called oral hairy leukoplakia. This appears as a white, warty area on the side of the tongue and on the cheeks inside the mouth. It may be caused by a virus.

Doctors have tried to establish whether any of these conditions can predict which patients are more likely to develop AIDS. Some studies have suggested that the appearance of oral hairy leukoplakia and oral thrush indicates that the person is at greater risk of progressing to AIDS. An earlier indicator may be the development of shingles, however. Shingles results from reactivation of the herpes zoster virus (also called varicella), which causes chickenpox in childhood. The infection can remain latent in nerve cells, flaring up again when immunity is low. A study in New York of homosexual men infected with HIV found that about a quarter of them developed AIDS within two years of having shingles. Four years after shingles, almost half had developed AIDS, and over a quarter had died from AIDS. The man's risk of subsequently developing AIDS rose if the shingles was severe and painful and if it occurred on the face or neck. In this group of men, doctors diagnosed both oral thrush and oral hairy leukoplakia, on average, just over one year after the attack of herpes zoster. These researchers concluded that eight years would be about the longest incubation period between zoster and AIDS. By adding another two to seven years for the period between the development of antibodies to HIV and development of herpes zoster, they added, the risk of AIDS developing after HIV seroconversion must continue for at least ten to fifteen years.

Some people infected with HIV experience a rather different pattern of disease. Instead of developing characteristic infections, in conjunction with falling numbers of T-cells, some individuals instead suffer neurological symptoms. Nobody knows what determines the path of disease, although there are some indications that some strains of the virus have a greater tendency to infect the nervous system than others.

The neurological abnormalities suffered by people with AIDS are grouped together under the term AIDS dementia complex or AIDS encephalopathy. AIDS dementia complex is included in the new definition of AIDS which came into effect in September 1987. The first neurological symptoms to appear may include forgetfulness, lack of concentration and apathy. There may be an inability to initiate and control movements. Changes in behaviour may also occur. These neurological symptoms are caused by HIV attacking the brain and nervous system. Eventually, full dementia, similar to that which occurs in Alzheimer's disease, may develop. Incontinence, weakness, paralysis and inability to coordinate movements may occur. The person may become agitated, or withdrawn and mute.

Estimates vary as to what proportion of people with AIDS suffer from AIDS dementia complex. One group of American researchers has estimated that two out of three people with AIDS have significant symptoms by the time that they are close to death, with more suffering neurological abnormalities detectable only by special tests. One British researcher has put the figure much lower, at one in four. Most authorities are agreed, however, that there is no evidence at present to suggest that people who are infected with HIV but who remain physically well are at any higher risk of abnormal behaviour than the rest of the population. Fear of neuropsychological abnormalities is therefore no justification for denying employment to people infected with HIV.

When doctors first began to recognize that many patients with AIDS also developed mental disturbances, they initially thought that these symptoms might be due to the brain infections and tumours that some people with AIDS develop, or to psychological effects. Yet research has shown that HIV itself is to blame, even though it does not commonly infect nerve cells. Many studies have now confirmed that, in many AIDS patients, it is possible to isolate HIV and viral components from the brain and the cerebrospinal fluid, which bathes the tissues of the central nervous system. In some patients, the amount of virus isolated from the brain and cerebrospinal fluid is far greater than that present in the blood.

Postmortem examinations of the brains of people who had suffered from AIDS dementia showed that the tissue of the brain had shrunk. Under the microscope, researchers saw characteristic abnormalities. In some individuals, small groups of inflammatory cells appeared throughout the brain. Other patients had no inflammation, but spaces had appeared in some parts of the brain. Researchers also often found abnor-

120

mally large cells with many nuclei which they called 'multi-nucleated giant cells'. These cells seem to resemble the white blood cells in laboratory cultures that fuse together when infected with HIV (see p. 103). Before long, several teams of researchers had identified the infected cells in the brain as monocytes and macrophages. Other workers also suggested that the 'multinucleated giant cells' probably started out as macrophages, too, because of similarities in their structure.

Exactly how HIV enters the brain and causes dementia and other neurological symptoms is unclear. Researchers have put forward several theories and these are summarized in figure 10. One of these theories holds that HIV first infects the monocyte in the bloodstream. The infected cell passes across the blood–brain barrier – the tightly linked cells that keep the bloodstream separate from the fluid that bathes the central nervous system – and into the brain. Two things might then happen. First, the infected cells might release toxic chemicals. These substances might damage the nerve cells and the glial cells, which protect the nerve cells and manufacture the insulation around their fibres. Or, these toxins might attract inflammatory cells which carry out the damage themselves.

A second possibility is that the infected monocytes might affect the cells of the blood–brain barrier, so altering the permeability of the barrier. Such a change would alter the delicately balanced environment of the central nervous system, upsetting the function of the nerve cells.

Another theory is that HIV may be able to infect glial cells. Some researchers have found that HIV can attack these cells under laboratory conditions. In addition, investigators have found evidence that HIV can, on rare occasions, infect nerve cells. But it is still not clear to what extent such infection accounts for the malfunctions of the nervous system in people with AIDS.

One further proposal is that viral proteins released by infected monocytes could interfere directly with the function of nerve cells. In support of this theory, some researchers have shown that part of the envelope glycoprotein of HIV is similar

121

to a natural chemical called neuroleukin. Neuroleukin, a protein which is found in human skeletal muscles, brain and bone marrow, prolongs the life of embryonic nerve cells in laboratory cultures.

In the absence of neuroleukin, embryonic nerve cells grown in the laboratory tend to die rapidly. If researchers add neuroleukin, however, the cells are far more likely to grow and develop. Another substance, called nerve growth factor, has a similar effect on the cultured cells.

Some researchers have added HIV to cultures of nerve cells supported by either neuroleukin or nerve growth factor. They found that HIV consistently suppressed the growth of the nerve cells supported by neuroleukin, but did not affect those cells grown in nerve growth factor. After further tests, they concluded that the viral envelope protein, gp120, was able to inhibit the activity of neuroleukin, but not that of nerve growth factor. Subsequent analysis of the sequences of the amino acids, the small molecules that make up proteins, showed some similarities between the sequences of neuroleukin and gp120. In addition, a short sequence of amino acids which corresponds to the sequence common to both gp120 and neuroleukin can also block the ability of neuroleukin to support the growth of nerve cells.

The scientists concluded from their results that the viral envelope protein may compete with neuroleukin for binding to nerve cells. Those cells to which gp120 binds probably die sooner, and this could account for the neurological abnormalities of AIDS.

There is one more facet to this interesting theory. Neuroleukin is also produced by T-cells that have been activated by an antigen. In this case, neuroleukin has the function of stimulating B-cells to produce antibodies. Perhaps gp120 also interferes with neuroleukin's function in activating B-cells. Such interference could, of course, account for the strange behaviour of B-cells in AIDS. It might even be the primary role of this sequence of amino acids to sabotage the role of B-cells. If this is so, the researchers concluded, the brain may be an 'innocent bystander' in AIDS. It may be affected purely by

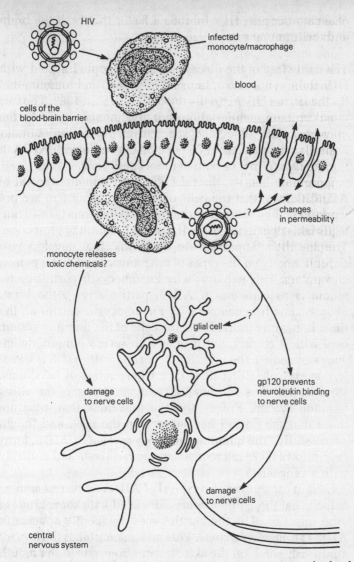

HIV

infected
monocyte/macrophage

blood

cells of the
blood-brain barrier

changes
in permeability

monocyte releases
toxic chemicals?

glial cell

gp120 prevents
neuroleukin binding
to nerve cells

damage
to nerve cells

damage
to nerve cells

central
nervous system

Figure 10. AIDS and the brain. Scientists are not sure which of
these theories may account for the dementia and other neurological
effects that some people with AIDS develop.

chance – because HIV inhibits a factor that both the brain and the immune system use.

The final stage of the disease for many people infected with HIV is the syndrome of unusual infections and tumours that doctors in the US originally dubbed 'AIDS' in 1982. The two most common manifestations are pneumonia caused by the microorganism *Pneumocystis carinii* and the tumour Kaposi's sarcoma. About 80 per cent of people with AIDS in the US have either or both of these conditions.

To immunologists, the infections and tumours typical of AIDS indicate that the cells of the immune system are not working as they should. Various microorganisms take advantage of this deficiency in the individual's immune protection. The so-called 'opportunistic infections' that develop will depend largely on the types of microorganisms that a person encounters. This explains why *Pneumocystis carinii* pneumonia is so common in AIDS, particularly in the West. People come into contact with *Pneumocystis carinii* all the time: in healthy individuals, the cells of the immune system deal with it readily, but people with severe immunodeficiency succumb to the infection. Someone with AIDS is therefore at risk of falling ill with a whole range of infections. Viruses, parasites and fungi all take advantage of the ailing immune system. Frequently, the infections that arise are those that the person has suffered in the past, and fought successfully. The immune deficiency present in AIDS, however, allows these microorganisms to reactivate and multiply with a vengeance.

Certain cancers are also typical of AIDS. Some researchers believe that these tumours are associated with some kinds of viral infection. The tumour that most frequently appears in AIDS is Kaposi's sarcoma. This malignancy takes the form of a purplish patch on the skin. It can also occur in the mouth and throughout the gut. In the US, Kaposi's sarcoma used to be rare – fewer than three cases per million men occurred every year. Yet, by the late 1980s, Kaposi's sarcoma was 2,500 times more common in young single men in the US than it

was in 1980. People with AIDS who develop Kaposi's sarcoma without suffering many opportunistic infections may
do better than those with pneumonia, for example.

Other tumours common in people with AIDS include lymphoma – a type of tumour which arises in lymph nodes – and
cancers of the mouth, tongue, bowel, rectum and anus. Some
studies have found that men with AIDS who had anal warts
also had a high risk of developing cancer of the anus.

In Africa, the range of infections and tumours is similar,
although HIV wasting syndrome – known as 'slim disease' –
may be relatively more common. The opportunistic infections may also appear with differing frequencies. Tuberculosis, for example, may be more commonly associated with
AIDS in Africa than it is in the US and Europe. Pneumocystis
pneumonia is less common in Africa.

Prompt diagnosis and treatment of opportunistic infections
and other problems will often return someone with AIDS to
a relatively good state of health. In between bouts of illness,
the person is often able to return to work and lead a normal
life. Much interest has been expressed, particularly by groups
of people with AIDS in the US and Europe, in the role of
diet, lifestyle and psychological attitude in influencing the
course of the disease. Many people with AIDS gain a great
deal of support and an improved sense of well-being from
such measures.

One of the factors that makes a diagnosis of HIV infection
particularly difficult to cope with, however, is that no one is
sure what proportion of HIV-infected people go on to develop
AIDS. According to estimates by the World Health Organization, between 10 and 30 per cent of HIV-infected people
will probably develop AIDS over a period of five years, and
20 to 50 per cent will develop other symptoms and illnesses
related to HIV infection. By 1988, many researchers were
saying that, in all likelihood, the majority of people infected
with HIV would eventually develop AIDS.

Any attempt to estimate the average incubation period –
from the time of infection to AIDS – is bound to be difficult
because many people do not know when they were first

exposed to the virus. Studies of particular groups of people – those infected via contaminated blood transfusions, for example – in which the date of transmission is known, have to be treated with some caution because the way in which the virus enters the body may influence the incubation period.

Nevertheless, scientists have studied data from the US on people who had received infected blood. By July 1988, there were over 1,700 cases of HIV infection from this cause in the US. The researchers found that the length of time that it took such people to develop AIDS varied according to their age and sex. On average, it took females almost nine years to develop AIDS from the time of infection, whereas it took males only between five and six years. Patients older than fifty-nine and younger than five developed AIDS more quickly. Those in the older age group took, on average, five and a half years to develop AIDS. Young children, on average, developed AIDS in just under two years.

It is difficult to draw firm conclusions from such a study, however. The researchers warned that no one knows how many people received infected blood transfusions in the days before health authorities screened donated blood for antibodies to HIV. So we cannot know what proportion of individuals infected in this way will eventually develop AIDS. In addition, it may not be possible to apply these results to people who became infected via sexual activity, for example. The researchers also emphasized that there was no way of telling how pertinent these figures were to the developing world, where people are exposed both more frequently and to a larger range of bacteria, viruses and parasites.

Doctors know with rather more certainty how long someone is likely to live once they have AIDS. About one in five is still alive after three years. The length of survival seems to depend on which particular condition the individual develops. People with *Pneumocystis carinii* pneumonia survive, on average, for about a year, although improved drug treatment is helping to prolong life. Those with Kaposi's sarcoma have a slightly better outlook, living for two to three years after diagnosis.

126

One encouraging breakthrough has been the development of tests which can predict which people infected with HIV are more likely to develop AIDS. One of these tests detects viral antigen – more specifically, the protein thought to reside in the core of the virus, called p24. This protein appears in the blood for a brief period at around the time that some infected people experience a short illness resembling glandular fever or influenza, before antibodies appear. Then, as the person develops antibodies to p24, the antigen disappears (see figure 11). Later on in the course of the disease, the situation reverses again. People start to lose the antibody to p24. As levels of this antibody drop, p24 antigen starts to reappear. One theory to explain these observations is that as replication of the virus increases during the later stages of infection, the amount of viral protein in the blood goes up. By forming complexes with the antibodies to p24, the antigen mops up the antibodies, thus accounting for their loss from the blood. (One hitherto unexplained oddity about this test, however, is that according to several reports, the level of antibodies to p24 does not decline in African patients as they progress towards AIDS.)

Doctors in the US have used a test for this viral antigen to diagnose early HIV infection in four previously uninfected homosexual men who had symptoms such as fever, rash, sore throat and aching joints and muscles. Normally, it is difficult to identify this initial illness as HIV infection because other viruses can cause similar symptoms and antibodies to HIV have not yet developed. In these four patients, tests for antigen were positive. All of them subsequently developed antibodies to HIV. So the test for antigen can allow doctors to diagnose infection with HIV at an earlier stage.

Research also suggests that people who keep producing antibodies to p24 are more likely to remain well than those who lose these antibodies and in whom antigen reappears. Loss of p24 antibodies and reappearance of p24 antigen is associated with a greater risk of progressing to AIDS. One study concluded that about half of all infected patients will probably develop AIDS within two years of the reappearance of viral antigen. In a second study, of HIV-infected men, most

127

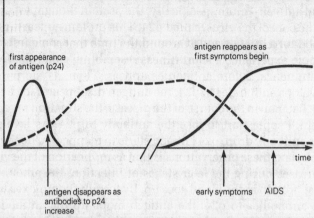

first appearance
of antigen (p24)

antigen reappears as
first symptoms begin

time

antigen disappears as
antibodies to p24
increase

early symptoms   AIDS

Figure 11. The viral protein p24 appears in the blood soon after exposure to the virus. Then, as antibodies to p24 develop, p24 itself disappears. Some research suggests that when the p24 protein reappears in the blood, at around the time that antibodies to p24 disappear, this signifies increasing viral replication, and a greater risk of developing AIDS.

of those without viral antigen in their blood remained free of symptoms. Those with viral antigen, however, were twenty times more likely to develop AIDS than those who were antigen-negative. The length of time that the man had had antigen in his blood did not seem to influence the outcome: antigen appeared between five and eighty-two weeks before the diagnosis of AIDS.

At the time of writing, the antigen test is available mainly to research scientists, but it will probably become more widely used in medical practice in the future. Doctors will be able to reassure patients who are doing well, and keep a close check on those at greater risk of developing severe infections. The test may also play a key role in the development of new drugs. If p24 antigen disappears in all the patients given a new drug, this might suggest that the drug is preventing viral replication. Such an objective means of assessing the action of a new drug would be far more accurate than asking patients how they feel and counting the number of infections they suffer. The antigen test will, it is hoped, greatly help doctors to establish whether a drug is effective or not, speeding up the process of evaluating new therapies.

Chapter 9

PATHS OF SPREAD

The spread of HIV is not inevitable. We have enough information now to prevent the virus spreading without check. But this strategy relies on changing people's behaviour, which is difficult to accomplish. Until scientists succeed in their struggle to develop a vaccine, which may take many years, the only way to control the epidemic will be to prevent the virus from spreading along its various routes of transmission – sexual intercourse, contact with blood and from mother to child.

It is interesting to contemplate how, after observing the first cases of AIDS in the US, doctors worked out the ways in which the virus passes from one person to another. In the US, as in many developed countries, AIDS first appeared in highly specific groups of people. If coughs, sneezes, handshakes, kissing and other types of casual contact had spread the virus, a completely different pattern of infection would have emerged, with cases appearing at random throughout the population.

Studies of who was affected allowed scientists to draw conclusions about what activities *can* spread the virus. Yet it is not such a simple matter for a scientist to say conclusively that a particular activity will *not* transmit HIV. Doctors and scientists will only go as far as to say that there is 'no sound evidence' for transmission by a certain route, that transmission is 'exceedingly unlikely' or that there is 'an extremely low risk' of the virus being passed on. Some people feel concerned by such cautious advice. In the real world, however, it is important to see such minute risks for what they are: unlikely. People who drive their cars to work every day, for example, have a small but definable risk of being killed or seriously injured in a traffic accident. No statistician would tell a group of car drivers – some of whom probably increase their chances of a serious accident by driving after drinking alcohol – that they are at no risk of an accident. Risks such as these are part of everyday life, whatever anyone does to try and reduce them.

There are parallels with the risks of becoming infected with HIV. During normal social contact with someone infected with HIV, there is, for all practical purposes, no risk of transmission of the virus. Under certain circumstances, however, it is necessary to take precautions in order to avoid possible infection. Some of these measures, such as screening of donated blood, are carried out by public-health authorities. Others, such as the wearing of a condom during sexual intercourse, are the responsibility of the individual.

There are times when people's fear of infection leads them to take protective measures where none is necessary. Such overreaction often stems from ignorance. Even people well versed in the evidence for and against a particular means of transmission can find it difficult to overcome their fear of such an unfamiliar disease. However, the basic research and observations on which scientists have based their advice on how HIV is and is not transmitted are revealing.

It is possible to isolate HIV from blood, semen, vaginal secretions, saliva, tears, breast milk, synovial fluid (which lubricates some joints) and amniotic fluid (the fluid that surrounds the baby in the womb). Just because it is possible to isolate the virus in the laboratory, however, does not mean that the fluid concerned is capable of transmitting the infection. There are several reasons why not. The concentration of virus may be too low; the body surface that the fluid comes into contact with may not include cells susceptible to infec-

131

tion; and there may be natural defences which stop the virus from attacking the new host.

There are three main ways in which the virus that causes AIDS can be passed on. These are sexual intercourse, contact with infected blood and from an infected mother to her baby.

During sexual intercourse, HIV can pass from man to man, from man to woman and from woman to man. There have also been one or two reports of transmission between two females as a result of sexual contact. Although AIDS first appeared among homosexual men in the US, all the evidence suggests that any type of penetrative sexual intercourse – anal or vaginal – can transmit the virus. In parts of Africa, the main means of transmission is via conventional heterosexual intercourse. Chapter 13 discusses in more detail what is known about heterosexual transmission.

The infection probably passes from a woman to a man when the virus, which can appear in vaginal secretions, enters the man's bloodstream via tiny abrasions on his penis. Some researchers are also trying to find out if HIV can directly infect the cells on the surface of the penis. Transmission from a man to another man or to a woman is easier to explain, for normal semen contains many T-helper lymphocytes, the type of white blood cell that HIV infects. One infected cell may harbour thousands of viruses. If the man has any other sexually transmitted diseases, he will have even greater numbers of T-cells and macrophages in his semen.

Interestingly, research has also shown that semen can suppress the function of the cells and molecules of the immune system in the recipient. This observation ties in well with the fact that homosexual men who practise receptive, as opposed to insertive, anal intercourse are often at greatest risk of HIV infection. In addition, sperm can act as antigens in the recipient, thus activating lymphocytes and macrophages. If the recipient is already infected with HIV, activation of these cells could set off viral replication. Together, these findings explain why some doctors recommend that people who are already infected should avoid further exposure to semen.

Avoiding sexual contact is, of course, important for people

who think that they may be at risk of catching the virus or of passing it on to their partners. The use of a condom during sexual intercourse helps to avoid the transfer of body fluids.

For homosexuals, it is clear that the most risky behaviour of all is unprotected receptive anal intercourse. A large study in several cities in the US, the Multicenter AIDS Cohort Study, monitored about 2,500 homosexual men for six months to see whether it was possible to identify which types of behaviour were associated with the development of infection. Within this group, there were 220 individuals who had practised neither receptive nor insertive anal intercourse during the period of the study. None of these men developed antibodies to the virus. In contrast, over 10 per cent of the 548 men who had had receptive anal intercourse during the period of the study did develop antibodies to HIV. Another group of 147 men reported having receptive oral intercourse with at least one partner, but not receptive or insertive anal intercourse. None of this group developed antibodies either. This observation, together with several similar studies, seems to suggest that there is a lower risk of transmission of HIV via oral-genital contact.

The study concluded that anal intercourse was the principal route of infection. The researchers said: 'A prudent course would be to stop anal intercourse entirely.' Other researchers, more pragmatically, have recommended that if it is not possible to avoid anal intercourse, the next best thing is to use a condom, together with a water-based lubricant, in order to prevent the transfer of body fluids. A condom will not eliminate the risk of transmission altogether, but it will greatly reduce it.

As far as heterosexuals are concerned, the virus can be transmitted by conventional vaginal intercourse. Anal intercourse between a man and a woman may, of course, also transmit HIV, but there is no evidence to suggest that anal intercourse is necessary for heterosexual transmission. Again, a condom will make sex safer if there is any risk that one or other partner is infected.

The second means of transmission is via blood. Doctors first identified this route in the West because some haemophiliacs began to develop AIDS. As discussed in Chapter 6, haemophiliacs need to take factor VIII to help their blood to clot. Many thousands of blood donors contribute to each batch of factor VIII, so haemophiliacs became vulnerable to HIV infection very early on in the epidemic. The development of a method of heat-treating factor VIII so that any viruses present are killed – and, more recently, the introduction of factor VIII manufactured synthetically – has greatly reduced the risks to recently diagnosed haemophiliacs in most developed countries.

People who have received contaminated blood in transfusions have also become infected. This mode of transmission is still a problem in many parts of Africa, where facilities for screening donated blood remain sparse. In the West, this method of spread is now extremely rare. American authorities began to screen donated blood in 1985. In Britain, all blood for transfusion is tested for antibodies to HIV. In addition, the blood transfusion service asks people in high-risk groups not to give blood. The only risk from a blood transfusion in countries where blood is screened is that someone might have given blood after becoming infected with the virus but before developing antibodies. The chances of receiving such contaminated blood are minute, however. In Britain in 1987, the blood transfusion service put this risk at one in five million. To put this figure in context, about half of the people who receive blood transfusions die within two years as a result of the injuries or illness that made a transfusion necessary in the first place.

In countries where the supply of sterile needles is plentiful, and needles are used once and then thrown away, there is no risk of catching HIV from injections or from giving blood. In some parts of the world, however, needles are scarce and may be reused for several people. Even though this practice ought to be avoided, many countries do not have the resources to pay for disposable needles and syringes. Some researchers have suggested that this route of transmission might partly account for the spread of the infection in Africa. Injections are commonplace in many parts of Africa, whether prescribed by doctors or by traditional medical attendants. Some ethnic groups also still practise scarification rituals. Conceivably, the instruments used to produce the scars on the skin could spread infection. Researchers have yet to establish precisely the role of exposure to unsterile needles or other instruments.

While it might be theoretically possible to become infected with HIV following ear-piercing, acupuncture, electrolysis and tattooing, no cases have been reported of infection by these routes. Of far greater concern in the West is the spread of HIV infection among people who inject drugs such as heroin. In some areas, for example Edinburgh in Scotland, over half of the drug users have antibodies to HIV. Drug users are at risk of becoming infected with HIV if they share a needle with someone who already has the virus. People can avoid spreading the virus by this route by using a clean needle and syringe, and not sharing needles with others.

As well as blood, donated organs and skin and bone grafts can carry HIV. There have been a few cases documented of people who became infected in this way, but infection by this route is very rare. Except in extreme emergencies, doctors now test organ donors for antibodies to HIV before carrying out a transplant or graft.

The third main method of transmission is from mother to child. An infected woman may pass the virus on to her child during pregnancy, at birth or with her breast milk during breast-feeding. In the West, information on the risks of passing on the virus during pregnancy or at birth is hard to come by because so few heterosexuals are infected. One study, in Edinburgh, of children born to women who are intravenous drug users, found that the mother passed on the infection to her child in about 50 per cent of cases. Scientists in Africa, however, have suggested that the risk may be lower, around 25 per cent.

Researchers from Project SIDA (SIDA is French for AIDS) in Kinshasa, Zaïre, and colleagues from the US, studied women attending hospital in Kinshasa. Almost 6 per cent of 6,000 pregnant women tested for HIV antibodies were seropositive. About half of the seropositive women had AIDS. The researchers tested seventy children born to infected mothers for a type of antibody which would suggest that the children were also infected. (Some types of antibodies can cross the placenta but their presence does not mean that the child is infected with the virus.) Only seventeen (24 per cent) of these seventy babies were positive in this test.

Seven months later, 18 per cent of the babies born to infected mothers had died, compared with only 1 per cent of children born to seronegative mothers. The same study found that a woman was more likely to pass on the infection to her child if she had AIDS or severe disease related to HIV infection than if she was infected but had no symptoms.

This study does not take into account the potential risk of transmission from breast milk if the child escapes infection while in the womb or during birth. It is difficult to separate these risks from each other, but there have been a few reported cases where breast milk was the only possible source of infection. For example, researchers working in Kigali in Rwanda reported the cases of two children who may have become infected by breast milk. The first case was in a child born to healthy Rwandese parents. The mother lost a great deal of blood during the birth and had a blood transfusion – her first ever – a day later. The child fell ill at the age of ten months and died nine months later. She had antibodies to HIV. The mother had been breast-feeding her daughter. In the past, people have suggested that transmission of the virus might be possible if the mother had cracked nipples. But in this case there had been no nipple problems.

The mother began to fall ill about a year after the birth. She had antibodies to HIV, although her husband did not, and she denied having had sexual contact with anyone other than her husband. When the researchers traced the two people who had provided the blood for her transfusion, one of them was infected with HIV. The mother must have passed the virus on in her breast milk some time after the birth.

The second case reported by this group of researchers was almost identical. Such reports have led some researchers to suggest that banks of human breast milk should be pasteurized. This process inactivates the virus. But the doctors in Rwanda emphasized that their report should not discourage mothers from breast-feeding, even in countries where HIV infection is common, as breast milk is best for the baby.

As scientists have built up a picture of how HIV passes from person to person, they have also managed to identify situations in which transmission does not occur. There is no evidence to suggest, for example, that contact with saliva or tears from an infected person poses any risk. It is true that it is possible, in the laboratory, to isolate the virus from saliva and tears, but one study puts this observation into context. Researchers in the United States tried to isolate the virus from eighty-three samples of saliva taken from seventy-one homosexual men who had antibodies to HIV. Fifty of the men also gave samples of blood at the same time.

The researchers were able to isolate the virus from twenty-eight of the fifty blood samples, but from only one of the samples of saliva. This sample came from a man with pneumonia and other signs of severe disease. The culture of saliva began to show detectable signs of viral activity (the presence of the viral enzyme reverse transcriptase) only after twenty-one days, yet this man's blood sample showed evidence of viral activity on day three. The scientists concluded that the virus is present only infrequently in saliva; when it is present, it occurs in very small amounts. In addition, one study has suggested that there is some factor in saliva that prevents HIV from infecting cells.

The issue for most people is whether they can become infected by, say, drinking from the same glass as an infected person, by sharing facilities such as a toilet, or perhaps by shaking hands. The evidence that ordinary social interaction of this kind presents no risk to uninfected people comes from several studies of the household contacts of infected people. Doctors in the US tested 101 people who had lived in the same households as thirty-nine adults with AIDS. None of these 101 were sexual partners of the patients with AIDS, but all had lived with an infected person for at least three months, and, on average, for about twenty-two months. Most of the families were poor and lived in crowded conditions, sharing items such as toothbrushes, towels, plates and drinking vessels, as well as facilities such as beds, toilets and baths or showers. The study showed that only one of the 101 household contacts was infected with HIV – a child who had probably been infected via her mother at around the time of birth.

Figures from the Centers for Disease Control support these results. According to the CDC, except for sexual partners, no one in the families of more than 12,000 people with AIDS is known to have developed the disease. The CDC cited five other studies which have also failed to find any transmission of HIV to adults who were not sexual partners of patients with HIV infection, or to children who were not at risk of transmission at the time of birth.

Another reassuring study was carried out in France, at a boarding-school for over a hundred haemophiliacs, epileptics and diabetics. All the children shared dormitories, classrooms, swimming-pools, dining-hall and lavatories. At the end of three years, half of the haemophiliac children had developed antibodies to HIV as a result of receiving contaminated factor VIII to help their blood to clot. But none of the non-haemophiliac children had antibodies to HIV.

Some people have been concerned about whether it would be possible to catch HIV infection from public swimming-pools. In a properly maintained and disinfected pool, this is extremely unlikely. Any blood that did enter the water, from a cut on an infected person, say, would immediately be greatly diluted. In addition, chlorine kills the virus. Furthermore, if the pool were not properly disinfected, the risks of catching hepatitis B, meningitis or polio would be far higher than that of picking up HIV. There have been no cases to suggest that it is possible to become infected from a swimming-pool.

One unfounded theory which has caught the imagination of many people is the question of whether blood-sucking insects could transmit HIV from person to person, in the same fashion as mosquitoes spread malaria. There is a great deal of evidence against this idea. One of the most convincing observations is the pattern of spread of the virus. In Africa, malaria is more common in children than in adults, which suggests that mosquitoes bite children more often than adults. Yet children rarely have HIV infection, unless they were born to an infected mother, or are old enough to have caught the infection by sexual contact. HIV infection is also much less common in rural areas than in towns in Africa. If mosquitoes spread HIV, the opposite would be true. And in Africa, as in the US and Europe, studies have shown that people sharing the same household as an infected person have no increased risk of the disease, unless they are a sexual partner or a young child of the infected individual. As many researchers have said, it is an odd mosquito that prefers to feed on prostitutes and dislikes feeding on children.

Why should mosquitoes be able to transmit malaria but not HIV? When a mosquito takes a meal of blood from an infected person, the parasite that causes malaria enters the mosquito's salivary glands, where it multiples. When the mosquito feeds subsequently, it injects an anticoagulant — along with more malarial parasites — to keep the blood of its victim flowing. But, unlike the organism that causes malaria, HIV is unable to replicate in the cells of insects.

If HIV cannot survive in the mosquito, the only other way in which such blood-sucking insects could theoretically transmit the virus is mechanically: the insect's mouthparts would have to act as a tiny hypodermic syringe. Researchers have explained why transmission in this way is very unlikely. Although insects can transmit some viral diseases, in these cases the concentration of virus or of infected cells in the blood is very high. By contrast, only one in 10,000 lymphocytes is likely to be infected with HIV — and, as described earlier, many people with AIDS have very low numbers of lymphocytes anyway.

Thomas Monath, a virologist with the Centers for Disease Control, has studied in some detail the issue of whether mosquitoes and other blood-sucking insects can transmit HIV. The CDC sent researchers to a town called Belle Glade in

Florida, after allegations that the town had an exceptionally high incidence of AIDS, comparable to that in the areas of highest prevalence in the United States, San Francisco and New York City. Some scientists suspected that mosquitoes were to blame. But the researchers found that high-risk behaviours such as use of intravenous drugs, prostitution and multiple sexual partners were common in the town. In addition, most cases were in young adults; there were no cases in children or elderly people. So there is no evidence here that mosquitoes can transmit HIV.

Monath has managed to 'infect' another blood-sucking insect, the bedbug, with HIV. The virus can survive in blood that remains on the insect's mouthparts or in its gut. But the chances of a bedbug transmitting the infection are minute, for the following reasons. Bedbugs can transmit two other diseases, called equine infectious anaemia and bovine leukosis. Both of these infections are caused by retroviruses, the family of viruses to which HIV belongs. Yet in both cases, the amount of virus that appears in the blood of the infected horse or cow is very high. Monath says that for a bedbug to transmit these diseases, the blood must contain over one million viral particles per millilitre. The blood of people with AIDS, however, usually contains only about ten viral particles per millilitre.

Another factor to consider is how much blood the insect can hold on its mouthparts. The volume of blood that a bedbug can transfer is of the order of one fifteen-thousandth of a millilitre. Monath calculates that the amount of blood on a hypodermic needle is about 140 times the amount of blood on the mouthparts of a bedbug. Yet, of the many health care workers who have accidentally stabbed themselves with a contaminated needle, only a few have become infected.

The Centers for Disease Control has been closely monitoring the incidence of cases of HIV infection in health care workers. In March 1988, just over 5 per cent of people with AIDS for whom information on occupation was available were health care workers – close to the proportion of the

140

American workforce employed in this field. This suggests that being a health care worker does not greatly increase someone's risk of becoming infected with HIV. Nevertheless, there is obviously a risk involved in handling blood from patients who may be infected with the virus, notably when accidents occur that bring a patient's blood into close contact with the health care worker. Such accidents usually involve either so-called 'needlestick' accidents – a stab with a needle which has been used to take blood from a patient – or splashes of blood or other body fluid into or on to the eyes, mouth or skin of the health care worker.

By the end of December 1987, the Centers for Disease Control had enrolled in a study more than 1,100 health care workers who reported that they had been exposed to blood or other body fluids from patients infected with HIV. Out of 870 people tested who had had needlestick accidents or cut themselves on something sharp in the presence of blood from an infected patient, only four became infected with HIV. All of them had reported exposure to blood rather than other body fluids such as urine or saliva. (One of the four, however, was not tested until ten months after the accident. This person also had a heterosexual partner who was infected with HIV, and may have been infected as a result of heterosexual transmission.)

In addition, more than a hundred people reported accidents in which blood, saliva, urine or other body fluids from infected patients had splashed either into their eyes or mouth, or into an open wound, or on to skin which was not intact (due to chapping, for example). None of them became infected with HIV.

Two other large surveys in the US are also studying HIV infection in health care workers. By April 1987, the National Institutes of Health had tested more than a hundred health care workers who had had needlestick injuries, as well as almost 700 health care workers, some of whom had had several accidents, in which their skin, eyes or mouth had been exposed to blood from patients infected with HIV. None of them became infected with the virus. Other studies in the

141

US, Britain and Canada, involving more than 450 health care workers who had had similar accidents, have found none who subsequently became infected with HIV.

There have, however, been reports of six people in the US and four in other countries who became infected with HIV following either a needlestick injury or exposure of skin or mucous membrane (such as eyes or mouth) to contaminated material. This material was blood from an infected patient in all cases except one. The exception was a laboratory worker who had been working with concentrated virus and had cut himself or herself on something sharp.

Another six health care workers were also found to be infected with HIV following accidents at work. One of them was also a laboratory worker who had been using concentrated virus. Investigations failed to identify other factors that would have put these people at risk of HIV infection, but, in these cases, the development of antibodies following the accident was not documented. No one knows, therefore, exactly when these people became infected.

The *Morbidity and Mortality Weekly Report*, reviewing this evidence, concluded that the risk of someone becoming infected following a needlestick accident involving blood from a patient infected with HIV is less than 1 per cent. In other words, out of a hundred health care workers who stab themselves with a needle contaminated with blood from an HIV-infected patient, only one is likely to become infected with the virus.

The report points out that health care workers are increasingly more likely to encounter patients infected with HIV as the epidemic spreads. All health care workers should therefore stick closely to guidelines designed to reduce the risk of transmission when caring for patients, the report concludes.

Some people who work in the health services, including doctors, have called for all people seeking medical care to be screened for antibodies to HIV. Yet many medical authorities believe that such demands are misguided. Apart from the problems of needing to obtain consent for such tests, screening of this kind would not be an effective way of protecting

142

health care workers. In many situations, especially emergencies, the result of the test would not be available rapidly enough for staff to act on the information supplied. And a negative result might provide a false sense of security: the person might be infected but not yet have developed antibodies. In places where there is a high incidence of infection with HIV, such as San Francisco, health care workers already routinely take precautions to prevent transmission of blood-borne viruses with all patients. Some authorities argue, however, that in areas where few people are likely to be infected with HIV, such a high level of protection is not warranted. The practical and ethical considerations involved in caring for patients who may be infected with HIV are among the many problems that society has yet to solve in relation to the spread of the human immunodeficiency virus.

Chapter 10

QUEST FOR A CURE

Infection with the human immunodeficiency virus poses an exceptionally difficult problem for scientists who hope to cure the disease. The virus integrates its own genetic material into the cells of its host. To destroy those foreign genes would mean eradicating all infected cells. In the early days of the epidemic, this option might have seemed feasible. HIV infects the blood cells known as T-helper lymphocytes. These cells have a limited lifespan, and the bone marrow continuously produces new blood cells to replace the old ones. Perhaps, scientists wondered, it might be possible to wipe out a whole generation of T-helper cells, eliminating the virus in the process.

Then it became clear that HIV also attacks other cells, including cells in the brain. The prospects of ever ousting the virus from the body receded further. Even if scientists could control the damage that the virus causes to the immune system, the brain could still act as a reservoir of infection from which fresh virus could spring. It is also now certain that many of the neurological symptoms of AIDS and HIV infection are the result of the effects of the virus on the brain and nervous system. In order to have any influence on this aspect of the disease, antiviral drugs would have to penetrate the blood-brain barrier, the tightly-linked cells that line the blood vessels in the brain, and preserve the delicately controlled environment which nerve cells in the brain need.

Although there is little prospect of ever being able to eliminate the infection from the body, this does not exclude the possibility of developing a treatment. The history of medicine suggests, however, that progress in treating AIDS is more likely to come about by a series of increments rather than in a single breakthrough. The discoveries of penicillin and subsequently of other antibiotics are notable exceptions.

There are three main approaches to the treatment of AIDS and HIV infection. The first is the prevention, early diagnosis and treatment of opportunistic infections. Secondly, there is the possibility of devising therapies which attempt to restore the immune system to its normal state. The third strategy is to develop drugs which interfere with the replication of HIV.

The prevention, early diagnosis and treatment of opportunistic infections can, in many cases, prolong the lives of people with AIDS, and their quality of life. The success of this approach obviously depends on the availability of affordable medical care and suitable diagnostic facilities. One example of how successful this strategy can be is the treatment of pneumonia caused by the microorganism *Pneumocystis carinii*. Some people with AIDS suffer repeated attacks of this pneumonia. Two antibiotics are effective against the infection, but both have side effects that demand a change of drug in up to half of all patients. Doctors in San Francisco decided to try a method that would deliver the drug direct to the lungs, using a device which turns the drug into a very fine spray which the patient inhales. The drug, pentamidine, stayed where it was needed – in the lungs. As a result, unpleasant side effects on other organs were avoided. Regular use of the spray can also prevent further attacks of this pneumonia.

Many other infections common in AIDS are readily treatable, provided that they can be diagnosed. Antifungal drugs are effective against thrush, for example, and effective antiviral drugs are now available for the treatment of infections caused by herpes viruses and cytomegalovirus. Development of new drugs effective against the common opportunistic

145

infections would nevertheless help to improve the quality of life, as well as prolong life, for people with AIDS.

Attempts to boost the immune system have not, so far, met with great success. In most cases, the techniques involved are also expensive, impractical or both. One strategy has been to give antibodies taken from people who are infected with HIV, but still well, to people who have developed AIDS. Some researchers believe that the symptomless phase of the disease is the result of an immune response by the infected person. When this response fails, AIDS develops. So if people with AIDS receive antibodies from people without symptoms, so the reasoning goes, these might help to reverse the process.

There are some indications that this technique can be helpful, particularly in children with AIDS. Such children have no immunity to the usual childhood diseases. The defects in their immune systems seem to interfere with their ability to make antibodies in response to new infections. Some researchers believe that this therapy cuts the number of infections that develop in affected children. However, this treatment is expensive and provides no long-term solutions for the patient.

Another technique which doctors have tried is transplantation of bone marrow. The bone marrow manufactures all the different kinds of blood cells, including T-cells. Researchers hoped that a bone marrow transplant would boost the number of T-cells. But apart from the difficulty of finding suitable donors, the effect is short-lived: the virus infects the transplanted cells, too. This method might offer some hope in the future, if used in conjunction with a drug effective against HIV.

Scientists believe that the defects in the immune system in AIDS are not only due to a shortage of T-cells but also result from abnormal behaviour of the T-cells that are left. In particular, the T-cells do not produce chemical messengers known as cytokines in the normal way when they are stimulated by an antigen. Cytokines influence the behaviour of other cells, especially macrophages, the large mobile cells that have the task of trapping, engulfing and eliminating

146

microorganisms. Some cytokines attract macrophages. Others inhibit macrophages from leaving once they have reached the site of infection. Some cytokines, such as the interferons, enhance the activity of other cells of the immune system. So, researchers postulated, perhaps it would be possible to compensate for defects in the production of these chemicals by giving someone doses of cytokines. Most of the studies carried out so far, however, have been on very small groups of patients, which makes it difficult to draw firm conclusions about the results.

One related strategy is to try to boost the number of T-cells with chemical messengers naturally found in the body. One such substance has the awkward name of 'granulocyte-macrophage colony-stimulating factor' or GM-CSF for short. Researchers in the US reported that GM-CSF could increase the number of white cells circulating in the blood. In laboratory tests, it stimulates the immature cells of the bone marrow to divide and develop, and boosts the ability of macrophages to kill tumour cells. Researchers have also shown that GM-CSF can inhibit the replication of HIV in infected cells grown in the laboratory.

In a small study in which patients with AIDS received an infusion of GM-CSF for a period of two weeks, the numbers of their white blood cells rose. After the infusion was stopped, however, the white cells returned to their previous levels. Studies of this substance are still continuing. Advocates of GM-CSF suggest that it might help patients who cannot tolerate drugs such as zidovudine because of the effect on the bone marrow. (GM-CSF may also prove useful for people with immunosuppression caused by conditions other than AIDS, such as those receiving radiation therapy or taking toxic drugs for the treatment of cancer. They may be able to tolerate larger, more effective doses without suffering the ill effects of damage to the bone marrow.) Other researchers, however, advise caution. They warn that a substance that stimulates T-helper cells may also activate the virus, thus speeding the course of the disease.

Many companies and researchers are racing to develop

147

other therapies that they hope will boost the immune systems of people infected with HIV. Trials of so-called 'immune regulators' are continuing both in the US and Europe. Most of these studies involve only small groups of patients, and it is difficult at the time of writing to draw firm conclusions about their results.

The third strategy for treatment of HIV infection and AIDS is to develop drugs that will interfere with the replication of this retrovirus. In order for such a drug to be widely used, it must be cheap and able to be taken by mouth. As it would probably have to be taken for the rest of the patient's lifetime, it should be without toxic side effects. To combat the neurological effects of HIV, the drug would need to be able to pass through the blood–brain barrier. It would also have to interfere with the virus in such a way that the virus could not circumvent the action of the drug by mutating.

Scientists know a great deal, and are finding out more all the time, about the life cycle of HIV (see p. 96). Instead of making it more difficult to design drugs to interfere with the virus, however, the intricacies of its replication provide a multitude of targets for potential drugs. The very complexity of the virus may prove to be its downfall.

One obvious target for a drug against HIV is the viral enzyme reverse transcriptase. This enzyme is unique to retroviruses. Without it, the virus cannot replicate. During the mid-1980s, researchers investigated several drugs that appeared to inhibit reverse transcriptase in laboratory tests. These drugs included suramin, which was originally developed in the 1920s to treat sleeping sickness (trypanosomiasis) in Africa, and HPA-23, which contains the chemical elements antimony and tungsten. It was the hope of treatment with HPA-23 that prompted Rock Hudson's flight to Paris in July 1985.

Trials of these drugs in small groups of patients with AIDS have failed to demonstrate any clear benefit. Toxic side effects have been a problem with HPA-23 and studies of suramin provided no evidence that the drug could stop the virus

148

replicating in patients. Neither drug is currently being enthusiastically investigated for the treatment of AIDS.

A third drug, phosphonoformate (foscarnet), was also thought to act by inhibiting reverse transcriptase, although later tests have shown that it is only poorly active against the virus. Small studies of this drug in patients infected with HIV came up with some promising results. Others have reported severe side effects. But even if this drug were proved to be effective against the virus, several problems would still remain. For a start, it has to be given by a constant intravenous infusion, direct into the blood stream. No oral preparation is available. Secondly, it does not penetrate the blood–brain barrier well.

The strategy of inhibiting reverse transcriptase can be successful, however, as zidovudine, formerly known as AZT, has proved. Zidovudine (trade-name Retrovir) started life with the cryptic label 'Compound S'. Scientists had first isolated it in 1964 during a search for drugs that would be effective against cancer. Twenty years later, the American pharmaceuticals company, Burroughs Wellcome, during a trawl for compounds that could combat the virus that causes AIDS, found that Compound S could inhibit retroviruses in the laboratory.

The compound was azidothymidine or, to give it its full chemical name, 3'-azido-3'deoxythymidine. Its correct generic name is now zidovudine – an essential change to avoid any confusion with the immunosuppressant drug azathioprine. Tablets of azathioprine carry the initials 'AZT' and it would be extremely unfortunate if people were to mistake this drug for zidovudine.

Zidovudine is a member of a class of drugs called nucleoside analogues. Nucleosides are the chemicals that make up the backbone of the DNA molecule. Each nucleoside contains a sugar as well as one of the four bases that code for the genetic information in DNA. Zidovudine is an analogue of the nucleoside thymidine (see figure 12). Both contain the base thymine, but zidovudine contains a modified sugar. (This bears an azido group, which led other companies earlier to

149

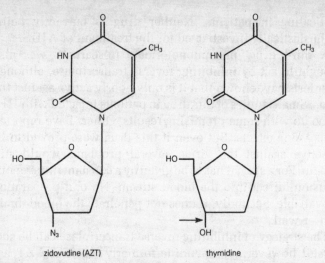

Figure 12. Zidovudine (left) is very similar in structure to the naturally occurring nucleoside thymidine (right). Where thymidine has an -OH group, however, zidovudine has a −N₃ group.

reject the compound as a possible antiviral drug, because of fears that it could be a potential carcinogen.)

When HIV infects a human cell, the viral enzyme reverse transcriptase controls the formation of viral DNA, using viral RNA as a template. The DNA molecule grows as reverse transcriptase adds new nucleosides to it. Unlike thymidine, however, once zidovudine has attached itself to the growing DNA chain, the next nucleoside cannot join it (see figure 13). So zidovudine blocks the process of DNA synthesis by terminating the chain.

All cells have an enzyme, called DNA polymerase, that controls the normal manufacture of new molecules of DNA by addition of nucleosides. There is some evidence that reverse transcriptase accepts nucleoside analogues more readily than DNA polymerase. This preference explains why zidovudine affects the replication of HIV in infected cells to a greater degree than it does in the replication of uninfected cells. Zidovudine and similar drugs inhibit viral replication at

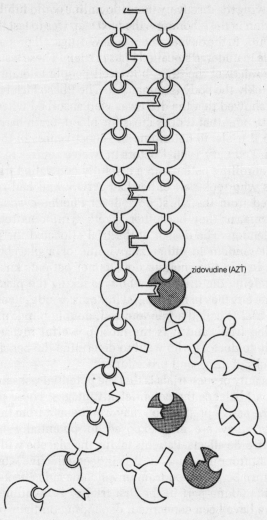

zidovudine (AZT)

Figure 13. The difference in the structure of thymidine and zidovudine means that once zidovudine has been incorporated into the DNA molecule, the next nucleoside cannot join the growing chain.

concentrations ten to twenty times lower than those at which they would kill normal human cells.

Following the discovery that zidovudine could inhibit viral replication in the laboratory, the next step was to test the drug on patients. In the development of new drugs, all preparations first have to undergo so-called Phase I trials. These tests establish the safety of the drug, how well people tolerate it, and how quickly the body eliminates it. The Phase I trial of zidovudine showed that the drug was well absorbed when taken by mouth, and that it does cross the blood–brain barrier.

Phase II trials, to determine the effectiveness of the drug, began in February 1986. Doctors in twelve centres in the US started enrolling patients in a carefully controlled trial. The patients who took part either had AIDS, and had recently recovered from their first episode of *Pneumocystis carinii* pneumonia, or they had other severe symptoms related to HIV infection. The design of the trial allocated the participants at random to either zidovudine or a placebo preparation. In addition, neither doctors nor patients knew who was receiving the drug and who was taking the placebo, to eliminate any bias in reporting symptoms or side effects. This type of trial is called a 'randomized, double-blind, placebo-controlled trial', and it is the most powerful investigation available to doctors who want to determine the benefits and drawbacks of drugs and procedures.

The beauty of such trials is that the potential risks for those taking part balance the potential advantages. Those patients taking the active preparation may well benefit from the drug. However, they are also exposed to potentially harmful unknown side effects. Patients taking the placebo will derive no benefit from the drug – if it is indeed effective – but they will in turn be protected from unwelcome side effects.

Patients taking part in the first trial of zidovudine might therefore have been concerned, depending on their point of view, either that they were not receiving a treatment that they perceived might be helpful to them, or that they might be suffering unacceptable side effects from a powerful drug of unproven efficacy. With this anxiety in mind, the National

Institute of Allergy and Infectious Diseases in Bethesda, Maryland, set up a group of six people, independent of both the manufacturers of zidovudine, Burroughs Wellcome, and the researchers carrying out the trials, to monitor the results. This group, called the Data and Safety Monitoring Board, reviewed the results as they came through, first in August 1986 and again in September.

On 18 Sepember 1986, the board recommended that, on ethical grounds, the trial should no longer be placebo-controlled. In other words, patients who had previously been taking the placebo should in future receive zidovudine. Far more people had died in the placebo group than in the group taking zidovudine.

Doctors from the twelve centres taking part in the trial published their final results in July 1987 in the *New England Journal of Medicine*. Of the 282 patients enrolled, 145 received zidovudine and 137 took placebo. After six months, only one patient had died in the group receiving zidovudine. By contrast, there had been 19 deaths in the group taking placebo. Forty-five individuals taking placebo had developed opportunistic infections, compared with 24 receiving zidovudine. In addition, the number of T-helper cells in the people in the treated group had risen.

By April 1987, after nine months of treatment, 6.2 per cent of the original group taking zidovudine had died. In comparison, out of the former placebo group, excluding those patients who were severely ill when they began treatment, and died within a few weeks, the mortality rate was 39.3 per cent. Burroughs Wellcome reported in June 1988 that 87 per cent of the patients taking part in the trial who had been allocated to treatment with zidovudine from the start were still alive one year after the attack of *Pneumocystis carinii* pneumonia which defined the diagnosis of AIDS in these individuals. After two years, the proportion still alive had dropped to 47 per cent. The company maintained in June 1987 that too few of the former placebo group were still alive at that stage to give a meaningful mortality rate for this set.

These results were impressive. Yet zidovudine has some

significant drawbacks. One is toxicity. The most serious side effect is often suppression of the bone marrow, causing anaemia. The rapidly dividing cells of the bone marrow are particularly sensitive to substances that interfere with DNA synthesis. In the trial described above, 24 per cent of patients receiving zidovudine developed anaemia, compared to 4 per cent of those taking placebo. 21 per cent and 4 per cent respectively in these groups needed several transfusions of red blood cells. In addition, those on zidovudine reported feeling sick or suffering aching muscles, insomnia and severe headaches more often than patients in the placebo group. Doctors involved with the trials warned, in the same issue of the *New England Journal of Medicine*, that '. . . the drug should be administered with caution because of its toxicity and the limited experience with it to date.' Other doctors who use zidovudine to treat patients with AIDS have reported that 40 per cent or more are unable to tolerate it after about six weeks because of anaemia. Other abnormalities of the blood induced by the drug also sometimes force doctors to reduce the dose or stop the drug altogether. Some doctors have also reported that the patient's condition can worsen when the drug is stopped, with neurological complications presenting a particular problem.

Some researchers have criticized the premature termination of the initial trial. They believe that the opportunity of finding out about the long-term effects of the drug, compared to a placebo, has been lost for good. Champions of zidovudine, however, say that this criticism speaks for itself. If the drug was no good, no one would be talking about its long-term side effects.

The second drawback is cost. In 1987, zidovudine was the most expensive drug on the market. A year's course for one person cost $10,000 or £7,000. In 1988, the manufacturers brought the price down, to around $8,000 for a year's course. Why is the drug so costly? The raw material for zidovudine is the naturally occurring nucleoside thymidine. Burroughs Wellcome used to obtain this compound from herring sperm, but the demand for zidovudine is now so great that the company buys synthetic thymidine from a contractor. It is often the rule that it is cheaper to make large quantities of a drug, but Burroughs Wellcome has found it difficult to scale up production of zidovudine. One reason, the company says, is that two of the steps in its manufacture are highly explosive.

Burroughs Wellcome has said that it spent about $80m on developing the drug and expanding facilities to manufacture it. The cost, the company said in 1987, was still rising because development and testing of new candidate drugs were continuing. Nevertheless, sales of zidovudine during the first half of 1988 totalled £40m.

Health services in developed countries are already finding it difficult to handle the demand for such an expensive drug. Some patients in the trial described had severe symptoms due to HIV infection, but had not at that time developed full-blown AIDS. The results suggested that zidovudine postponed the progression to AIDS in many of these patients. During the late 1980s, two large trials began to determine whether zidovudine can help to delay the onset of AIDS in people infected with HIV. One, which began in the US in 1987, expects to include 1,500 people. Another, hoping for the participation of 1,000 patients in Britain and 1,000 in France, started in 1988. If zidovudine is proved to be effective in delaying the onset of AIDS, the market for the drug could be massive. Yet, in the US, many insurance policies do not cover the cost of drugs. People who want zidovudine but cannot afford it have to seek medical treatment at public hospitals.

In Britain, the cost of zidovudine for the treatment of AIDS has already put a strain on resources. In 1988, most of the health authorities which cared for significant numbers of AIDS patients were in London. In some, the expenditure on zidovudine can take up as much as a third or more of their total annual budget for drugs. The government has given some authorities extra funds to help them to pay for the care of AIDS patients. However, if zidovudine is proved to be useful in delaying AIDS in those who have antibodies to the virus but no symptoms, thousands of people who may have been exposed to the virus but who currently choose not to be tested will want to find out if they are infected. In Britain, where in 1988 there were estimated to be up to 50,000 people infected, the National Health Service could have some very unpalatable decisions to make about who should receive treatment.

Zidovudine is just one of a family of drugs called nucleoside analogues. Researchers at the National Cancer Institute in Bethesda, Maryland, have already tested on humans a second nucleoside analogue called dideoxycytidine. In the laboratory, dideoxycytidine halts the replication of HIV at about one tenth of the dose required with zidovudine. Other nucleoside analogues under investigation include compounds called cyanodideoxythymidine, dideoxyadenosine and dideoxyinosine. Biochemists could produce many different compounds, all of which might be active against the virus, by adding different chemical groups to nucleoside bases.

In May 1987, doctors at four hospitals in the US began the first tests of dideoxycytidine in people. Within a couple of months, some of the people taking the drug began to complain of pains in their feet. The pains were caused by a condition called peripheral neuropathy. Fortunately, the pains disappeared in most patients when doctors withdrew the drug. Some participants also developed unpleasant skin rashes.

The investigators went on to test dideoxycytidine on another group of people, this time using lower doses. They want to find out what is the highest dose that they can use without causing side effects, and whether this dose modifies the course of the disease. Doctors also plan to test alternating therapy: one week on zidovudine followed by one week on dideoxycytidine, and so on. The theory is that such a regime might avoid the side effects that result from each of the two drugs given alone.

An interesting feature of zidovudine, dideoxycytidine and their relatives is the way in which they become active in the cell. In normal DNA synthesis, each successive nucleoside, in order to add itself to the growing chain of DNA, needs to be in a form known as a triphosphate. In other words, it has to have three chemical groups known as phosphates. Without these phosphate groups, the nucleoside cannot take part in the reaction that attaches it to the DNA. Zidovudine has to undergo the same process. Cellular, as opposed to viral, enzymes turn the drug into its active form, zidovudine triphosphate. (There is some evidence, though, that some types of cell cannot perform this step efficiently.)

The need for cellular enzymes to activate these drugs is a characteristic that researchers may be able to exploit in designing new drugs of this nature. Pharmacologists would like to be able to target the drug selectively on infected cells. This approach would avoid the problem of toxicity, where the drug unnecessarily poisons other tissues and organs. Researchers are trying to find mechanisms, specific to infected cells, which would selectively activate the drug. For example, the virus might induce novel enzymes in infected cells. Any drug that depends on cellular, rather than viral, enzymes for its activity also has the advantage that mutations of the virus are unlikely to lead to the virus becoming resistant to the drug.

Designers of drugs are trying to develop ways of inactivating reverse transcriptase. Researchers have already determined the sequence of amino acids in the enzyme. The next step is to work out the molecule's three-dimensional structure. To do this, scientists first have to prepare the chemical in the form of a crystal. Then they use X-rays to examine the structure of the crystal. Scientists at Wellcome's laboratories in Britain announced in 1987 that they had crystallized reverse transcriptase and planned to examine its three-dimensional structure. Unfortunately, the crystals that they had obtained by late 1988 were not well ordered enough to provide the required information about the molecule's structure. Wellcome's researchers therefore sent a crystallization experiment into space on the shuttle in late 1988. Better crystals form in space under conditions of low gravity, and the researchers hoped that crystals obtained in this way would provide the information they needed. Thus armed, their aim

157

is to design drugs that can inactivate reverse transcriptase, perhaps by binding to the part of the enzyme crucial to its activity.

There are, however, other vulnerable points in the life cycle of the virus. One ideal strategy would be to prevent the virus from binding to its target cell in the first place. There are several ways in which scientists might achieve this. One would be to develop highly specific antibodies that would block the CD4 receptor molecule. The consequences for the host's immune system are unknown, however, and some researchers believe that such a strategy could be dangerous. Antibodies which block the binding site on the viral envelope protein are another possibility. But this might be difficult, as the binding site seems to be hidden in a cleft in the protein.

A similar approach would be to block the entire viral envelope protein with another protein. This is the strategy behind a potential therapy which researchers in the US began testing on patients in the second half of 1988.

In late 1987 and early 1988, several companies reported that they had managed to produce quantities of the CD4 protein to which HIV binds, using techniques of genetic engineering. By inserting the genetic information for this protein into cells which were then grown in bulk, the companies were able to harvest large amounts of the protein. The resulting product is known as recombinant CD4. Doctors hope that when people infected with HIV take this substance, it will act as a decoy for the virus, mopping up free virus and preventing it from infecting cells. In 1988, a trial of recombinant CD4 began in three centres, involving about fifty volunteers with AIDS who would take CD4 for six months to determine whether it has serious side effects. If this trial is successful, the next step would be to give the protein to more volunteers in order to test its effectiveness in curbing the decline of the immune system. At the time of writing, results from the initial trial are not available, but many researchers have high hopes that recombinant CD4 will prove both safe and successful.

Other researchers are also investigating the possibility of developing a short stretch (or peptide) of CD4 which would

158

prevent HIV from infecting cells. Scientists in the US reported in 1988 that they had identified a peptide which would block the ability of HIV to kill cells in laboratory experiments. They believe that a peptide may be more useful than the whole protein, because it may be able to cross the blood–brain barrier, and may be more resistant to being broken down by the body's enzymes.

Another substance which seems to block the binding of the virus to its target cell is a drug called dextran sulphate. This is a compound containing both glucose and sulphur. It has been available in Japan for two decades for its action in reducing the clotting ability of the blood, and its ability to lower lipids in the blood.

Researchers have shown that dextran sulphate can prevent HIV from binding to T-cells. The drug was able to prevent the genetic material of HIV from becoming incorporated into the cells. Initial tests in people with AIDS suggested that dextran sulphate had some antiviral activity at doses that did not appear to be dangerous. In the drug's favour is the fact that it is available without a prescription in Japan; Japanese researchers say that there is extensive evidence that the drug has low toxicity and few side effects. By mid-1988, several centres in the US had begun clinical trials of the drug involving sixty volunteers. Results of these early tests were not available at the time of writing.

Drugs that prevent the virus from binding to the target cell will only be able to modulate the course of the disease at times when the virus is actively replicating. Such drugs should be able to prevent new viruses produced in the body from infecting fresh cells. It would also be useful, however, completely to prevent infected cells from producing new viruses. One way of doing this would be to interfere with the part of the virus's life cycle that takes place inside the cell. There are plenty of targets, although many of the possible strategies are still highly theoretical.

It may be possible, for example, to find substances that will prevent the virus from uncoating itself after it has entered the cell. Researchers in the US have already discovered compounds that will prevent picornaviruses (which cause diseases of the respiratory and gastrointestinal tracts, as well as polio) from uncoating. These compounds act by fitting into a cleft in the core shell protein of picornaviruses. These viruses do not have a fatty envelope layer as HIV does, but the compounds can pass through lipids, so this difference should not present too much of a problem. The researchers are now studying the core protein of HIV to determine its structure. The next step will be to try to design compounds that fit in a cleft of this protein, thus preventing the virus from delivering its genetic material to the cell.

Once the viral genetic material has inserted itself in the DNA of the cell, other strategies can come into play. HIV has quite a complicated system of regulating its own production. Three of its genes, known as *tat*, *rev* and *nef*, produce proteins which help to regulate the replication of the virus (see figure 14). The proteins produced by the *tat* and *rev* genes seem to be essential if the virus is to make any of its other proteins. The protein made by the *nef* gene downregulates the production of the virus's structural proteins, without which viral replication is impossible.

Any of these proteins could be useful targets for antiviral drugs. Researchers are studying the proteins to find out how they can inhibit them. It might be possible to do this by manufacturing short segments of protein that block the protein's active site. An alternative might be a short sequence of genetic building blocks which would bind irreversibly to the virus's genetic material, preventing the manufacture of the protein.

Researchers working in the US announced at the Fourth International Conference on AIDS, held in Stockholm in June 1988, that they had shown that a similar approach could work. They developed short modified sequences of DNA that bind to the *rev* gene. These sequences, called 'phosphorothioate oligodeoxynucleotides' or S-ODNs, were able to stop the gene's activity and so prevent the virus from replicating. The researchers reported that the sequences could not only prevent HIV from infecting normal T-cells but also inhibit the virus from reproducing in infected cells. Although this work

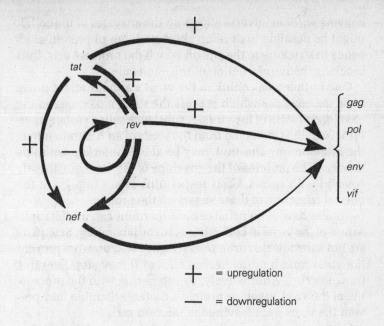

tat

rev

nef

gag
pol
env
vif

$+$ = upregulation

$-$ = downregulation

Figure 14. The current theory of how HIV regulates the production of its proteins. The proteins produced by the gag, pol and env genes are structural proteins. Without the protein derived from the tat gene, it is virtually impossible for the virus to make any of its other proteins. The protein from the rev gene downregulates its own manufacture – as well as that of the tat gene. Any of these genes could prove useful targets for antiviral drugs.

is encouraging, the scientists say that much more research will be needed before a therapy based on this approach will reach the stage of testing in patients.

Another vulnerable point in the life cycle of the virus might prove to be during the assembly of viral particles. For example, viral enzymes called proteases play an important role in cleaving large precursor proteins into smaller molecules which form the mature virus. The fact that a viral enzyme carries out this step, rather than one supplied by the host cell, suggests that human cells have no closely related enzymes. So it might be feasible for researchers to inhibit this enzyme without adverse effects on the enzymes of the cell. It might be possible to develop short stretches of protein analogous in structure to the site on which the protease acts, thus blocking the normal action of this molecule.

One further weak chink in the virus's armour might prove to be the enzymes which process the sugar molecules on the envelope protein of the virus. A substance called castanospermine, which is extracted from the seeds of an Australian tree, the Moreton Bay chestnut, may be able to interfere with this process. The proteins of the envelope of the virus are densely covered with sugars. Castanospermine seems to prevent the normal trimming of these sugars on the proteins.

Studies have shown that castanospermine can inhibit replication of the virus in cell cultures in the laboratory. Scientists are not sure how this drug works, however. It does not prevent the virus from binding to the cell, but it may stop the virus from entering. Alternatively, by interfering with the processing of the viral envelope proteins, castanospermine may prevent the virus from leaving the infected cell.

Castanospermine may be too toxic to use in patients. It may be possible, however, to design new drugs that act in the same way by analysing the action of castanospermine. Scientists have already begun to test several similar drugs.

This chapter has not so far mentioned several drugs which have, in recent years, attracted a great deal of publicity. In many cases, both scientists and companies, excited by initial results which they believed to be promising, have made announcements about the efficacy of drugs which later turned out to be without foundation. In some cases, companies seem to have paid more attention to ensuring that the stockmarket knew about their results than to informing the medical community. The motive, no doubt, was to boost their share prices. Other drugs have come to grief because the research on which the initial optimism was based was faulty. Hundreds of people are buying other drugs on the black market and taking them without any scientific proof of their efficacy.

Some drugs claimed to be effective in treating AIDS have

faded as rapidly as they arrived. For example, controversy surrounded the announcement that some researchers had discovered a short fragment of protein, called peptide T, which seemed to block the virus's ability to infect cells. Other scientists reported that they could not reproduce this work. Some researchers criticized the fact that some patients had already been given peptide T, despite the failure of several laboratories to confirm the initial results. Claim and counter-claim ensued. In late 1987, some of the original researchers announced that a trial of peptide T would take place in Los Angeles, to determine whether the substance was toxic and, eventually, whether it can influence the course of infection with HIV. Twelve patients were to take part. Some initial results from this trial were presented at the international conference on AIDS which took place in Stockholm in June 1988. One of the researchers said that the trial had proved that peptide T was safe. In addition, patients receiving peptide T had reported that they felt more vigorous and less tired. However, as members of the audience pointed out, the patients taking peptide T were not compared to those taking a placebo, so the 'improvements' cited may have been due to the 'placebo effect', where people taking a drug feel better simply because they have faith in the treatment.

Another drug initially thought to have some potential as a treatment for AIDS was fusidic acid. Laboratory tests of this drug, a proven antibiotic, appeared to show that it could completely inhibit the infectivity of HIV. Unfortunately, research published later showed that the lack of viral activity arose because the drug was, in fact, killing the cells in which the virus lived. A clinical trial in patients, carried out before this news became available, also found that the drug had no beneficial effect on patients with AIDS. Researchers now accept that fusidic acid has no role in the treatment of HIV infection.

Yet another contender in the late 1980s was ampligen. This was said to work both by inhibiting the virus in some way and by stimulating the immune system, by promoting the production of the chemical messengers called cytokines. Ampligen consists of special sequences of the genetic material RNA. Although RNA normally has only one strand of smaller molecules, in ampligen the RNA is double-stranded: it has two strands wrapped round each other.

Researchers initially tried using double-stranded RNAs to treat patients with cancer more than ten years ago. The theory was that it might be possible to harness the body's own defences against tumour cells. In these first trials, the patients suffered such severe side effects that doctors had to abandon this approach. Researchers then found that by modifying the RNA – the result was ampligen – they could eliminate the toxic effects. Later, they reported that ampligen could inhibit the replication of HIV in cells grown in the laboratory.

The next step was to see what effect ampligen had on patients with HIV infection. The initial results seemed promising. In June 1988, some of the researchers reported that ampligen seemed to be able to strengthen the body's immune system and suppress HIV in people infected with the virus. There was 'significant clinical improvement', doctors reported. As a result, a nine-month study involving 200 patients began. Yet by October 1988, the two companies supporting the trial withdrew from the project, on the grounds that there was no reduction in the rate at which patients taking ampligen were progressing to AIDS.

Ribavirin is another drug which has found little favour, with the medical establishment, at least. This drug is already licensed in several countries for the treatment of respiratory infections, caused by respiratory syncytial virus, in children. It is also effective in the treatment of viral diseases such as Lassa fever.

The Californian company which makes ribavirin, ICN Pharmaceuticals, says that the drug is also active against HIV. ICN claims that the drug works by selectively preventing the virus from completing copies of the genetic material RNA which carries the information necessary for the manufacture of viral proteins. Yet tests of ribavirin's activity in the treatment of HIV infection had not, by 1988, provided clear-cut results.

During 1987, ICN clashed with the Food and Drug Administration in the US, which had claimed that patients in a study supported by the company had not been randomized to placebo and treatment groups in an acceptable way. Specifically, patients in the placebo group seemed to be more ill than patients in the treated groups, which could account for the fact that more patients taking placebo died than patients taking one of two doses of the drug. A group of independent scientists and statisticians re-evaluated the study, however, and many of them said that ICN should be allowed to carry out further studies of ribavirin. In September 1987, the Food and Drug Administration agreed to allow the company to conduct further trials with the drug. Results of these studies are not available at the time of writing. However, British researchers who considered carrying out trials of ribavirin have reported that the drug has no effect on circulating viral antigen (see p. 127). If levels of this antigen fall, this is normally a good indicator that the drug has some action against the virus. Ribavirin, however, does not seem to have this effect.

Despite the lack of good evidence that this drug works, there is an organized black market in ribavirin over the border between California and Mexico. Gay pressure groups in California have provided detailed advice on how to obtain ribavirin and other drugs that are not available in the US but can be bought in Mexico. The safest strategy on returning through customs, the advice says, is to declare a personal supply of the drug.

Yet it seems unfortunate that many people have spent their time and energy on buying a drug which has no proven efficacy. An American pressure group called the National Gay Rights Advocates (see p. 167) has pointed out that in these circumstances, 'a person's use of the drug [ribavirin] is totally unsupervised, without any benefit to research in this country'. By the late 1980s, enough people had probably taken enough ribavirin to answer the question of whether this drug is effective against HIV many times over. Because these patients were not taking part in clinical trials, however, much potentially useful information has been lost.

People with AIDS are understandably desperate to try any

165

new therapy that offers some hope, in the absence of effective drugs approved by the medical establishment. Many people with AIDS, impatient with what they saw as the establishment's failure to speed up investigations into novel treatments, have turned to 'kitchen sink' recipes such as AL721. This substance, a mixture of natural lipids (fats) made from egg yolks, is a yellow oily liquid which can be taken spread on bread or in orange juice. The 'AL' stands for active lipid; the '721' represents the ratio of the three different lipids that the mixture contains. Eager to grasp the opportunity to take matters into their own hands, many gay pressure groups in the US and Europe organized themselves to obtain and distribute bulk supplies of the necessary ingredients.

AL721 is now so widely taken that it may prove impossible to evaluate scientifically. Once people perceive a treatment as useful and effective, it becomes very difficult for doctors to enrol patients into a randomized, placebo-controlled trials (see p. 152). Those who take part may be so concerned that they may not be receiving the active preparation that they may secretly take their own home-made version. This kind of action invalidates the results and makes analysis impossible. The blame for this state of affairs does not lie with the people who try to do something for themselves, however, for the progress of AL721 along the path of scientific evaluation has been painfully slow.

AL721 was discovered by researchers in Israel. They developed the substance because they found it could remove molecules of cholesterol from cell membranes. Those who advocate AL721 as a treatment for HIV infection suggest that it may work by changing the density of the fatty membrane of the virus, so that the envelope proteins which normally project from the surface of the membrane sink down into it, concealing the sites necessary for binding to the target cell. However, there is no scientific proof that AL721 has any efficacy in treating HIV infection. Doctors who wanted to test its effect on people with AIDS have been hampered by inadequate and intermittent supplies of AL721 from the manufacturers. The results of one trial were reported in Stockholm in

June 1988, however. Doctors in Germany said that patients given AL721 did very badly. In addition, cells taken from these patients had lost the receptor molecules such as CD4, without which these cells cannot function. Most medical authorities no longer consider AL721 to be a viable therapy.

Many people infected with HIV believe that the standard procedures for testing novel therapies are unnecessarily slow. If a disease inevitably kills within three years, sufferers are not going to be able to wait four years for new drugs to be tested. The families and friends of people with HIV infection, as well as the sufferers themselves, have become understandably angry and frustrated at the lengthy machinations of the regulatory bodies that control the approval of new drugs.

In the US, even changes in the Food and Drug Administration's regulations on new drugs for 'desperately ill' patients, in force since June 1987, do not seem to have improved matters. People have resorted to the courts to try to find out why there have been long delays in evaluating certain treatments. One pressure group, the National Gay Rights Advocates (NGRA), even tried to sue the heads of several American government departments for failing to act swiftly enough in developing new treatments. NGRA alleged that the Food and Drug Administration had accelerated testing and approval only for drugs developed or sponsored by the National Institutes of Health (NIH), a government body.

The lawsuit claimed: 'NIH concentrated its research into NIH-sponsored drugs, or into drugs developed by companies with which NIH or its researchers had developed special relationships, such as Burroughs Wellcome or Hoffman-La Roche . . . NIH ignored or seriously delayed consideration and testing of other promising drugs.' The Food and Drug Administration, the group alleged, applied more stringent procedures and requirements to drugs developed privately than it did to zidovudine. 'NIH's decisions,' the lawsuit continued, 'were affected by essential conflicts of interest, namely, royalty payments from manufacturers licensed to develop NIH-sponsored drugs.'

Public loss of confidence in the system in the US has already led to one state taking matters into its own hands. On 28 September 1987, the governor of California, George Deukmejian, signed an emergency bill to allow California to carry out its own testing and licensing of drugs. It would have been difficult for him to refuse, for the bill had wide support from politicans. The state Legislative Assembly had passed it by seventy-nine votes to nil, and the Senate by thirty-eight to nil. At the time, the state attorney-general, John Van de Kamp, said: 'This bill is the state of California's announcement that, in the face of an extraordinary medical emergency, business as usual just isn't good enough.'

The law means that California can test, manufacture and distribute experimental drugs within the state – provided that all raw materials come from within California. Some commentators believe that the result could be a black market in novel drugs over the border with California. Dubious manufacturers and suspect therapies could mushroom. A spokesman for the Food and Drug Administration, which denies that it is being too slow in testing new substances, warned that there may be dangers in approving new drugs too quickly. The state of Nevada, for example, licensed a compound called laetrile. People used this substance, which is highly toxic, to treat cancer, even though there is no evidence that it is effective.

Throughout the whole of the US, however, there is a growing demand for people to be able to obtain and take drugs that they think will help them against AIDS. In response to public pressure, the Food and Drug Administration announced in 1988 that it is legal for people to import drugs from abroad for their personal use. Frank Young, the commissioner of the Food and Drug Administration, making this announcement, told gay and lesbian activists that the policy was not new, nor limited to drugs against AIDS. The amount of drug may not exceed three months' supply for one person, and the person importing it may not sell it to anyone else. This ruling is meant to prevent the development of a black market. Although this means that people can import drugs not yet approved by the Food and Drug Administration, substances or so-called cures that the administration believes are fraudulent are still banned.

Young made his statement following controversy over the import of dextran sulphate, a drug freely available in Japan (see p. 159). Americans with AIDS had been making trips to Japan and bringing back as much of the drug as they could.

Some researchers have criticized this move on the grounds that it will make it more difficult to evaluate new drugs scientifically. Patients who suspect they may be given a placebo in a double-blind trial may also take other drugs available on the black market, to try to ensure that they obtain some benefit, somehow. Many patients are becoming reluctant to enter trials, because they fear they may receive only a placebo. This view ignores the fact that patients who receive a placebo are protected from any adverse side effects that may be associated with the active drug. The history of medicine is full of examples of therapies enthusiastically received that, when properly evaluated, turned out to do more harm than good. However, it is becoming clear that some people would be prepared to accept the risks of side effects if it meant a chance of receiving a drug which has at least some evidence to suggest that it may be effective. Researchers may find that if they fail to give thought to designing trials which are both acceptable to patients and scientifically sound, their patients will have gone elsewhere.

Chapter 11

TOWARDS A VACCINE

Scientists face a tough task in designing a vaccine to protect people against AIDS. If they were to draw up a list of characteristics that would make it exceptionally difficult to develop a vaccine against a particular microorganism, the chances are that the human immunodeficiency virus would meet most of those criteria. Frequently, as research has progressed, the goal of a vaccine against AIDS has seemed to recede rather than draw nearer. However, instead of being discouraged, many researchers feel that they now understand more clearly the problems that they have to tackle.

Perhaps the most daunting obstacle of all is that a vaccine against HIV would need to prevent completely the initial infection. If it did not, the virus would still be able to integrate its genetic material into cells and HIV would be irreversibly established in the body. A vaccine that failed to prevent this step, even if it could prevent the development of AIDS in those who later became infected, would be unlikely to be approved by the licensing authorities. Nor would such a vaccine be acceptable to the general public, although it might have a place in protecting those who are at high risk of infection. The long-term sexual partners of infected people, if still uninfected themselves, might consider taking such a vaccine, for example.

Most vaccines that protect against infectious diseases, however, need only *limit* the infection when the vaccinated person encounters the bacterium or virus concerned, rather than prevent it entirely. With the immune system primed by the vaccine to recognize the infectious agent, the immune response is rapid and effective. Antibodies and specialized cells produced by the immune system help to eliminate the foreign invader. The curiosity of HIV infection is that although the immune system seems to make all the right kinds of response that would normally effectively combat a microorganism, this virus remains unscathed. It persists in the body and the antibodies against it do not signify immunity. Doctors have never discovered anyone who appears to have recovered from infection with HIV with immunity to further attacks.

There are four main responses by the immune system aimed at eliminating microorganisms. First, there are neutralizing antibodies, produced by activated B-cells. By binding to the microorganism, neutralizing antibodies can help the body to eliminate the intruder. Secondly, the production of substances such as interferon can limit the spread of viruses to surrounding cells. A third mechanism is the activation of T-cells which can help to destroy cells infected with the microbe. Lastly, the immune system produces 'memory' cells of both the T and the B variety. These are ready to spring into action whenever the immune system encounters the same microorganism in the future.

The immune systems of people infected with HIV do, in fact, respond well to the virus. They produce neutralizing antibodies to its envelope protein, although, admittedly, these remain at low levels. They also produce cells, called cytotoxic T lymphocytes, that can kill cells infected with HIV. Finally, they produce antibodies that help other cells of the immune system, called killer cells, to eliminate infected cells. (This process is called antibody-dependent cell-mediated cytotoxicity, or ADCC.)

Why, if the body makes a good response against HIV, does the virus manage to persist and eventually cause AIDS? How can researchers design a vaccine to protect against HIV when

171

they do not know what kind of immune response is effective against it? Scientists will have to find the answers to these questions if they are ever going to achieve their goal of an effective vaccine against AIDS.

By the late 1980s, there were at least some theories to explain why the immune system fails to eliminate HIV. One is that the genetic material which holds the information for the envelope protein of HIV mutates very rapidly, many times faster than that of the influenza virus. Research on vaccines against influenza has shown that antibodies produced against one influenza virus may not recognize a second strain of the virus, thus failing to protect the individual against the second strain. The same principle applies to HIV. If antibodies produced against the virus could protect someone against infection, they may be effective only against the original viral strain which stimulated their production and not against others. Researchers have even isolated different strains of HIV from a single individual at different times after infection. The immune system must find it difficult to keep up with such a constantly moving target.

Another possible explanation for HIV's ability to evade the immune system is that HIV can spread from cell to cell. This may be significant at the stage of initial infection. Infected cells in a man's semen, for example, may enter the body of his sexual partner. The virus inside the cell is protected against the recipient's antibodies, particularly if the infected cell does not show any viral proteins on its surface. Even if there are viral proteins on the cell's surface, the recipient's cytotoxic T-cells, whose task it is to eliminate virus-infected cells, may be powerless against such an invasion. The cytotoxic T-cells of the recipient can recognize viral proteins on the surface of an infected cell only in conjunction with other proteins (called MHC proteins) normally found on the recipient's body cells. Unless the MHC proteins on the surface of the donated cell closely resemble the MHC proteins of the recipient, the recipient's cytotoxic T-cells will be unable to act. The infected cells will be able directly to infect the recipient's cells. Furthermore, once someone is infected with HIV, the virus can pass from cell to cell, completely evading the immune system.

The third theory depends on the fact that HIV grows not only in T-helper cells but also in macrophages and their immature forms, monocytes. Macrophages are able to engulf and destroy foreign microbes bound to antibodies. But with HIV, this may be the way that the virus enters macrophages. Once there, it may set up a silent infection which again evades the immune system.

Finally, there is a hypothesis to explain why immune cells capable of killing body cells infected with virus fail to complete this task. The reason may be that infected cells may reside somewhere in the body where killer cells cannot reach them. Two possible sites are the brain and central nervous system and the bone marrow. Infected cells in these so-called 'immunologically privileged' parts of the body may form a reservoir of infection.

The fact that none of these theoretical scenarios has been proved to take place demonstrates how little is known about the body's immune response to HIV. Designing a vaccine to protect against this virus will be difficult given the extent of this ignorance. For example, some researchers have suggested that, if it is true that most macrophages become infected as a result of engulfing virus-antibody complexes, then a vaccine which stimulates the body to make antibodies will be of little use. It could even be harmful, because it would spread the virus to the macrophages.

Despite these uncertainties, scientists are pushing ahead with work to determine which strategies they should use to induce immunity to HIV. If a vaccine is to prevent infection, it will have to stimulate the production of specific antibodies that will neutralize the virus. So the work of some researchers is aimed at trying to boost the levels of neutralizing antibodies to the virus to much higher levels than tend to occur in the natural infection. By the late 1980s, however, there was increasing emphasis on ways of priming the cells of the immune system to recognize and eliminate the virus. A vaccine that stimulated the production of appropriate cytotoxic

T-cells would control, rather than prevent, the infection. Many researchers believe that an effective vaccine would need to induce both antibodies and cell-mediated immunity in order to protect against HIV.

In developing a vaccine against a new disease, it is natural to turn to techniques which have worked for other viral diseases in the past. There are two tried and trusted methods. Killed vaccines are those based on viral particles which have been inactivated. These particles can no longer infect their host, but they are still capable of provoking an immune response that can protect their host against infection by the live virus. Secondly, there are the live attenuated vaccines. These contain live viruses which have been attenuated (weakened), sometimes by growing them for many generations in the laboratory. These vaccines infect the host without causing disease. The immune response that they induce can protect the host against subsequent infection with the virulent strain from which the vaccine was originally derived.

Vaccines based on these methods have helped to control diseases such as poliomyelitis, yellow fever, measles and rabies. Unfortunately, it is difficult to apply the same techniques to develop a vaccine against AIDS. It would never be possible to use a live attenuated vaccine because of the risk that the weakened virus could mutate and again become capable of causing disease.

Some researchers have not yet ruled out the possibility of using a killed vaccine to protect against AIDS, however. Doctors and scientists in California are investigating whether a preparation of inactivated HIV might delay the onset of AIDS in infected people. The logic behind this approach is that, if it is possible to stimulate an effective immune response at all, this response might be able to prevent those already exposed to the virus from developing AIDS.

Jonas Salk, of the Salk Institute in La Jolla, California, is leading the research. It was Salk whose pioneering work led to the development of a vaccine against poliomyelitis in 1954. This vaccine, like the preparation Salk is trying against AIDS, also consisted of whole inactivated viruses. Salk is collaborating with a company called the Immune Response Corporation, also based in La Jolla. This company is producing the inactivated virus, first by exposing it to gamma radiation and then by stripping it of its outer envelope proteins, replacing these with a layer of mineral oil.

At the international conference on AIDS, held in 1988, Salk told delegates that he and his colleagues, including Alexandra Levine from the University of Southern California, had inoculated nine homosexual men with the preparation. These men had severe symptoms of HIV infection, but not AIDS. The initial results, Salk said, suggested that the preparation can induce the production of antibodies and immune cells. Only one patient continued to lose T-cells after the inoculation, and there appeared to be no toxic effects. Salk said his next move would be to test the preparation on healthy people infected with HIV.

One reason for hope that this technique might work is that researchers at the University of California at Davis developed a similar vaccine several years ago which seems to protect monkeys against simian AIDS. Nevertheless, even if Salk's approach seems to work in healthy people infected with HIV, some scientists have reservations about the safety of inoculating healthy people with a preparation containing even the inactivated genetic material of a retrovirus.

Such considerations have forced researchers to investigate novel ways of making vaccines. Even before the need to develop a vaccine against AIDS arose, research was already in progress aimed either at improving existing vaccines or developing vaccines against diseases for which vaccines were not yet available. The most important finding from this research was that only one, or sometimes two, of the proteins of a virus was all that was needed to induce protective immunity against the live virus. This discovery opened up the prospect of new vaccines, based on just one or two proteins, which would have none of the disadvantages associated with vaccines consisting of whole viruses. Because these vaccines would be based on just a small part of the parent virus, scientists have called them subunit vaccines. The recent

175

development of techniques of genetic engineering also raised the possibility that, once researchers had identified the genes containing the information for the proteins required, they would easily be able to manufacture the proteins in bulk for use in a vaccine.

Scientists found, furthermore, that it was sometimes possible to identify short segments (peptides) of the protein which were responsible for its ability to provoke an appropriate immune response. Peptides are so small that chemists can synthesize them in the laboratory.

The new generation of vaccines that scientists are now developing – including many aimed at protecting against HIV and AIDS – is therefore based on identifying and manufacturing a component of a virus that will, on its own, induce immunity to the disease caused by that microbe. (The other half of the battle is to find an appropriate way of 'presenting' that protein or peptide to the immune system. Unfortunately, isolated proteins stimulate the immune system less effectively than the entire microbe. This is probably because the three-dimensional configuration of the protein changes once it is away from the confines of the parent virus. Techniques of presenting proteins to the immune system are reviewed later in this chapter.)

There are several different ways of manufacturing a single protein in bulk using genetic engineering, but the general principle is the same in each case. Once researchers have identified the gene containing the information for the required protein, they insert it into cells such as those of the bacterium *Escherichia coli*, a harmless microorganism that lives in the gut. They then grow the cells, which are deceived into making the foreign protein as well as their own, in large vats. Finally, they purify the viral protein, which can account for as much as a fifth of the weight of the cultured cells.

Proteins manufactured in this way will not be exactly the same as the proteins that appear in the intact virus. For example, some viral proteins are covered with sugars: scientists say that they are glycosylated. Proteins manufactured in *E. coli* are not glycosylated. If researchers require the protein to be glycosylated, they can achieve this by inserting the gene for the protein instead into yeast cells or mammalian cells (such as those from hamster ovaries), which do glycosylate the proteins they manufacture.

Another approach is to insert the gene for the required protein into a second virus. Vaccinia virus, which induces immunity to smallpox, is one obvious choice. Some researchers are also investigating the potential of another virus called adenovirus.

Vaccinia virus contains a large amount of DNA, not all of which the virus needs in order to replicate. Researchers have therefore replaced parts of the virus's vaccinia genetic material with genes from other viruses. These genes contain the information for proteins that induce immunity to particular diseases. The engineered vaccinia virus manufactures the foreign protein, which appears on its surface.

Apart from being a good way of manufacturing the desired protein, many researchers also believe that this is an effective way of 'presenting' the protein to the immune system. Because the protein appears on the surface membrane of the vaccinia virus, they reason, it should resemble its natural appearance on the surface of the virus from which it was derived. It should thus stimulate the immune system more effectively than the isolated protein would. So, in this case, there is no need to isolate the protein from the virus which manufactures it. The engineered vaccinia virus would itself comprise the vaccine. Furthermore, one option would be to inactivate the engineered vaccinia virus in order to produce a killed vaccine. Some researchers believe that this is a useful approach when dealing with proteins from dangerous viruses – such as the rabies virus, for example.

A second virus which scientists have used in the bulk manufacture of proteins for vaccines is of a type known as a baculovirus. Like vaccinia virus, this virus does not need all of its DNA in order to replicate, and it is possible to replace some of the DNA with genes containing the information for the required protein. The baculovirus normally infects insects. It is easy to grow either in cultures of insect cells or in caterpillars. It is also an efficient method of manufacture. The protein, which has to be purified, can make up a significant proportion of the weight of the fully grown caterpillars or cultured cells – far more than in genetically engineered bacterial, yeast or mammalian cells.

Once scientists have quantities of the appropriate protein available, the next step in developing a vaccine is to devise a way of 'presenting' that antigen to the immune system. Purified proteins manufactured by techniques of genetic engineering only rarely have the same ability to provoke an immune response as they do in the intact virus. To compensate for this deficiency, scientists combine the viral antigen with a substance that enhances the immune response to it. Such substances, which are called adjuvants, appear to 'flag' the viral antigen to the immune system, although little is known about how they affect the immune system.

In most countries, only two adjuvants, aluminium hydroxide and aluminium phosphate, are licensed as safe enough for use in humans. But many researchers are working to develop improved safe adjuvants, as well as novel ways of presenting antigens. Some researchers, for example, believe that it is important to present the antigen in a regular array on a membrane – much as it would appear on its parent virus.

Researchers have proposed several ways of achieving this. One may be by manufacturing the protein in a vehicle such as vaccinia virus, as explained above. A second possibility is to use a 'pseudovirus'. Researchers in Britain, from the University of Oxford and a company called British Biotechnology, have made these by manipulating the DNA of yeast cells and the genetic material of the virus to which they wish to design a vaccine. The viral and yeast proteins derived from the engineered genetic material combine to produce particles which look just like viruses under the electron microscope. Injected into animals, these particles can stimulate an immune response directed against the viral protein included in the pseudovirus. The animals appeared to suffer no toxic side effects.

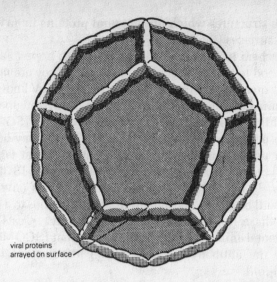

viral proteins
arrayed on surface

Figure 15. ISCOMS – the name is short for immunostimulatory complexes – have viral proteins arranged on their surface. ISCOMS are about the same size as viruses.

The researchers, Susan Kingsman, Alan Kingsman and Keith Gull, said that they planned to combine genes from HIV with yeast DNA in order to make a candidate vaccine against AIDS. In 1988, they said that a trial of the vaccine in humans could take place 'any time within the next two years'. But their first step will be to test the method by incorporating different proteins from the feline leukaemia virus (also a retrovirus) in a range of pseudoviruses and determine whether these preparations protect cats from infection with the feline virus.

Another possible means of boosting the immune response to a viral protein is called the ISCOM. The name stands for immunostimulatory complex. To make ISCOMs, researchers mix the viral protein on which they are basing the vaccine with a substance called Quil A, which comes from the bark of the Amazonian oak, in the presence of a detergent. Under these conditions, ISCOMs form naturally. They are small, cage-like structures which present viral proteins in an array on their surfaces (see figure 15).

Researchers in Glasgow, led by Bill Jarrett, hope to adapt this method to make a vaccine against HIV. They are manufacturing quantities of the envelope protein of HIV known as gp120 in insect cells infected with a genetically engineered virus. This protein will then be inserted into the ISCOMs. Some researchers are concerned that ISCOMs may be too toxic for use in humans. However, Jarrett says that tests in apes and monkeys over two years have shown that ISCOMs are safe. He hopes that ISCOMs bearing HIV's envelope protein will be able to boost neutralizing antibodies to a level where these provide effective immunity. Tests on experimental animals, he says, have shown that ISCOMs can improve the antibody response to a particular antigen a hundred-fold.

A very different approach, and one which many researchers believe holds a great deal of promise, is based on an existing vaccine against poliomyelitis. There are two types of vaccine against polio. One is the Salk vaccine, mentioned on p. 175, which consists of killed viruses. The other, the Sabin vaccine, is much cheaper and has the advantage that it can be taken by mouth, on a sugar lump. The Sabin vaccine is based on live attenuated viruses. It is extremely safe but, very rarely, paralysis can follow vaccination. Researchers at Reading University in England therefore began to study how they could make the vaccine safer.

The Sabin vaccine is a mixture of three strains of poliovirus. One is extremely safe, but the vaccine has to include the other two strains as well, in order to induce good all-round immunity to all three types of poliovirus. The scientists at Reading, led by Jeffrey Almond, identified small sections of the poliovirus which are crucial in stimulating the production of neutralizing antibodies. They then used genetic engineering techniques to alter the safest strain of poliovirus. They replaced some of the antigenic regions with the corresponding antigenic sections from the third strain. The so-called chimaeric virus which resulted was then capable of inducing an immune response against the third strain.

Almond and his colleagues now hope to insert small sections of proteins from other microorganisms into the poliovirus, to make vaccines against the diseases caused by these microbes. One reason why scientists believe that this method could be successful if applied to HIV is that poliovirus is very good at inducing the body to produce antibodies at mucous membranes, such as the mouth, the lining of the gut and the vagina. This type of immune response could be very important in preventing the sexual transmission of the human immunodeficiency virus. By the late 1980s, the Reading group had already constructed chimaeric viruses bearing antigens from HIV. Encouragingly, some of these were capable of replicating normally.

Other novel delivery methods which scientists are investigating include encompassing the protein (or peptide) which invokes an appropriate immune response in membrane-bound vesicles (known as liposomes); attaching the protein to a solid base by a monoclonal antibody which binds specifically to the protein; and containing the protein in glass which can take from a few hours to many years to dissolve and release its contents. The latter method would be practicable only if the vaccine consisted of a stable substance, such as a small peptide, which would retain its biological activity over many months or years. Such a vaccine would circumvent the problems inherent in many traditional vaccines which require individuals to return for further injections at specified intervals – a requirement with which people in many countries find it difficult to comply.

Scientists have no shortage of methods to try in developing a vaccine against HIV and AIDS. But first they have to identify the appropriate proteins or peptides from the human immunodeficiency virus which invoke an appropriate immune response. This is no easy task, given the lack of knowledge about the human immune response to the virus. The proteins which researchers have tried as candidate vaccines have been selected without any real indication of their usefulness as components of vaccines. Most candidate vaccines have concentrated on the envelope protein of the virus, following the general rule that proteins on the surfaces of viruses stimulate the immune system of the host to produce neutralizing antibodies. The increasing interest in stimulating cytotoxic T-cells has led to at least one candidate vaccine based on a protein from the core of HIV – in line with the observation that, on the whole, proteins in the viral core stimulate the cells of the immune system.

Many candidate vaccines that have reached testing in human subjects are, on this basis, shots in the dark. Nevertheless, the results obtained from these trials provide useful information about the human response to antigens of HIV. The first trial began in 1987, when the US Food and Drug Administration authorized tests in humans of a vaccine based on gp160, the envelope protein of HIV. This vaccine is called VaxSyn HIV-1.

The company making the vaccine, MicroGeneSys of West Haven, Connecticut, is growing the gp160 in insect cells, using genetically engineered baculovirus (see p. 117). After purification, the protein is 'flagged' with an adjuvant in order to enhance the immune response to it. Previous research has shown that VaxSyn HIV-1 can produce high levels of antibodies to gp160 (and to its component proteins, gp41 and gp120) in experimental animals. According to a report published in 1987 in the *Journal of the American Medical Association*, tests suggested that these antibodies might have been capable of neutralizing the virus. When researchers added serum from the injected animals to cultures of human T-cells, along with HIV, the virus did not infect the cells. The animals' antibodies may have prevented the virus from binding to the T-cells.

During 1987, scientists from MicroGeneSys began the trial in collaboration with doctors from the National Institute of Allergy and Infectious Diseases in Bethesda, Maryland. They aimed to recruit more than 150 people, including homosexual and heterosexual men, and some women, into the trial. Only people who had negative tests for infection with HIV were eligible to participate, and all those accepted to the trial received counselling on how to avoid infection with the virus.

This trial aimed to establish the safety of the vaccine. Researchers also wanted to find out what kind of immune response the preparation induced. For the purposes of comparison, some of the participants in the trial received a placebo, and others received a vaccine against hepatitis B. In 1988, researchers reported that twenty people in the trial had developed an immune response to the vaccine. Final results from this trial were due in early 1989.

Many other groups are also working to develop vaccines based on the envelope proteins. For example, researchers with the biotechnology company Oncogen – a subsidiary of Bristol-Myers based in Seattle, Washington – have genetically engineered vaccinia virus so that it displays HIV's gp160 on its surface. The Food and Drug Administration approved the application to begin trials with this candidate vaccine in November 1987. By late 1988, doctors had injected twenty-eight volunteers (uninfected with HIV) with the preparation.

Tests to establish the safety of a third candidate vaccine in humans began in mid-1988 in Switzerland. The vaccine is being made by a company called Biocine, which is equally owned by the pharmaceuticals company Ciba-Geigy and the American biotechnology company Chiron Corporation. The preparation consists of an altered form of gp120, manufactured in yeast cells using techniques of genetic engineering. This protein is then combined with a 'novel adjuvant' which has been developed by Ciba-Geigy. Doctors at a hospital in Geneva are conducting the trial, which aims to compare two different doses of the vaccine. Control groups will receive adjuvant alone. Biocine expects similar studies to begin in the US by 1989.

The tests that have drawn most publicity, however, are those conducted by the French researcher Daniel Zagury. He inoculated himself in November 1986 with a vaccine based on vaccinia virus. This had been genetically altered to carry the gene for the envelope protein of HIV, from a strain of the virus called HTLV-3B. He suffered no apparent side effects and went on to vaccinate a small group of Zaïrean volunteers.

In early 1987, he reported his results in *Nature*. Tests two months after the initial inoculation showed that Zagury had developed neutralizing antibodies against HTLV-3B, but not to a second strain called HTLV-3RF. Zagury then looked for evidence of cell-mediated immunity. He found that both strains of the virus could cause cells of the immune system from his blood to divide and proliferate, although HTLV-3RF stimulated them less effectively. (The fact that the cells divided and proliferated suggested that they had been primed to recognize the virus.) Two of the other people whom Zagury had vaccinated had also developed significant levels of neutralizing antibodies against the HTLV-3B strain of HIV.

Later that year, at the Third International Conference on AIDS, held in Washington DC, the ballroom of the Washington Hilton was packed with delegates and journalists eager to hear Zagury's latest results. He told the conference that he had followed the initial inoculation with a booster injection. The booster consisted of 'disabled cells'. These cells had been removed from Zagury and the other vaccinated individuals, infected with the vaccinia virus containing the gene for gp160, inactivated, and then injected back into the same individuals. This procedure, Zagury said, seemed to make it possible to induce antibodies which would neutralize many different strains of the virus. After Zagury left – chased out of the Hilton by photographers and reporters – one of the other speakers appraised what he had said. Dani Bolognesi, of Duke University Medical Center in Durham, North Carolina, said: 'I think he's taken a step that has eluded us for some time.'

In April 1988, Zagury reported further results in *Nature*. He had followed the first booster of 'disabled cells' with second and third boosters of genetically engineered envelope protein (gp160). Zagury and his colleagues found that antibodies present in his blood were able to neutralize several different strains of HIV. The researchers found evidence that Zagury had developed a good cell-mediated response as well.

These results, the team concluded, showed for the first time that 'an immune state against HIV' can be obtained in humans. But the results did not, of course, offer any evidence that the vaccine can protect someone against HIV or AIDS. Furthermore, the technique that Zagury used is highly impractical for immunizing large numbers of people. Zagury and his colleagues said in 1988 that they were trying to mimic the effect of the vaccine using methods that were more practical for large-scale use. Nevertheless, Zagury said in June 1988 that he intended to start large clinical trials with the vaccine in the very near future. He believed it would be about two years before he knew whether the 'vaccine' worked.

The three candidate vaccines we have described all rely on some form of the envelope protein of HIV to induce an immune response. A fourth candidate vaccine, which also began clinical trials in 1988, incorporates a protein from the core of HIV instead. This preparation is based on a peptide (short segment) of the protein called p17, which some researchers believe lies just below the surface of the virus. The vaccine is called HGP-30, from the number of amino acids which the peptide contains. The peptide closely resembles a section of the p17 protein, which tends not to mutate. It is being synthesized chemically.

This vaccine was developed by an American company called Viral Technologies. By late 1988, the US Food and Drug Administration had not approved clinical trials with this preparation. However, British authorities agreed to let trials begin. Doctors organizing the trial planned to give the vaccine to about twenty-five volunteers, all of them already infected with HIV. Some research suggests that antibodies to p17 drop suddenly in infected people about to develop AIDS. As with Salk's killed vaccine, the aim is to find out whether boosting the immune response to HIV in infected people can delay the onset of AIDS. Viral Technologies said in 1988 that it anticipates being able to extend the trial to uninfected people at high risk of infection.

By the late 1980s, there was little to indicate which, if any, of these approaches might meet with success. None of these

185

candidate vaccines, at least in their present forms, is even remotely close to being tested to find out whether it prevents infection with HIV. Possibly, researchers will find that one of these methods does induce an immune response – but one that will have an effect only against strains of HIV very similar to the one from which the vaccine was derived.

The variability of the proteins which comprise HIV is one of the biggest obstacles to a vaccine against this virus. Yet some components of the outer envelope protein, for example, must stay the same in all strains of the virus. If the region where the virus binds to the T-helper cell were to mutate, the virus would no longer be able to attack its target. Studies of the protein gp120 have shown that there are a few sites where the sequence of amino acids remains the same in several strains of HIV, as well as in the virus which causes AIDS in monkeys, SIV. One or a group of these so-called 'conserved' regions must form the binding site. (A group may be involved because the protein folds, perhaps bringing three or four different stretches of the protein together to form the binding site.)

Many researchers believe that blocking the binding site of the virus is the best strategy of all. Intensive research has already begun to try to map the entire envelope protein of HIV in order to identify which parts are concerned with binding. In one study, for example, researchers have manufactured eighty-six different peptides of the protein gp160. Each peptide is fifteen amino acids long, and overlaps with its neighbours on either side, so that every part of the protein is represented twice. By injecting each peptide into rats, the researchers will be able to produce and isolate a series of antibodies which recognize adjacent sites on gp160. By checking to find out which antibodies can prevent the virus from binding to its target cell, the scientists will then be able to work out which parts of the protein are involved in binding.

If researchers do manage to identify such a peptide, antibodies against which seem to block the viral binding site, this peptide might form the basis for a vaccine. Scientists would just need to choose which would be the best method of pre-

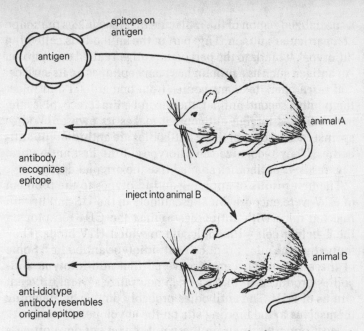

epitope on
antigen

antigen

animal A

antibody
recognizes
epitope

inject into animal B

animal B

anti-idiotype
antibody resembles
original epitope

Figure 16. Anti-idiotype antibodies are antibodies against anti-bodies. If you inject an antigen into animal A, the animal makes antibodies against that antigen. If you then purify those antibodies and inject them into animal B, this animal recognizes them as foreign and makes its own antibodies against them. Some of these antibodies are anti-idiotype antibodies: they resemble the original antigen.

senting this antigen to the immune system, out of all the methods outlined earlier in this chapter.

Some British and American researchers are also closely scrutinizing the binding site of the envelope protein with a different aim in mind. They are probing the potential of what some leading scientists believe is one of the most exciting approaches to a vaccine: 'anti-idiotype antibodies'. These antibodies may also prove effective as a therapy for people who are already infected with the virus.

An anti-idiotype antibody is an antibody to an antibody (see figure 16). What makes each kind of antibody unique is a specialized region of the molecule that recognizes the shape of a particular antigen. This part of the antibody is called the 'idiotype'. It binds to the part of the antigen called the epitope. An antigen such as a protein has many epitopes on its surface.

If researchers take antibodies from one animal and inject them into a second animal, the second animal recognizes the antibodies as foreign antigens. It makes its own antibodies against them. Some of these antibodies are anti-idiotype antibodies. They recognize the idiotypes of the first antibodies. The result is antibodies shaped like the original epitope.

The first results of applying anti-idiotypes to the problem of HIV were encouraging. Researchers in the US and Britain injected mice with antibodies against the CD4 receptor on the T-helper cell – the molecule to which HIV binds. They found that the mice produced anti-idiotype antibodies. Some of these scientists then discovered that anti-idiotype antibodies produced in this way can neutralize several different strains of HIV. The antibodies probably do this by attaching themselves to the binding site on the envelope protein.

Most importantly, from the point of view of developing a vaccine, they found that these anti-idiotypes could block the binding of both AIDS viruses, HIV-1 and HIV-2, as well as the related monkey virus, SIV. Work by researchers in London also suggests that the binding site on all three viruses is highly conserved. In other words, the molecules that form the binding site are the same in many different strains.

During the late 1980s, further work was in progress to try to map the binding site more precisely using a series of monoclonal antibodies that recognize different epitopes within the binding site. (Monoclonal antibodies are produced by genetically identical cells – clones – manufacturing quantities of a single type of antibody, which can then be purified.) Scientists may find that a single anti-idiotype antibody will not block binding effectively. A pool of several anti-idiotypes, each recognizing different sites, may be better at preventing the virus from binding to the T-cell.

This work may prove highly useful in designing a vaccine. Yet it may also be possible to employ similar strategies as a

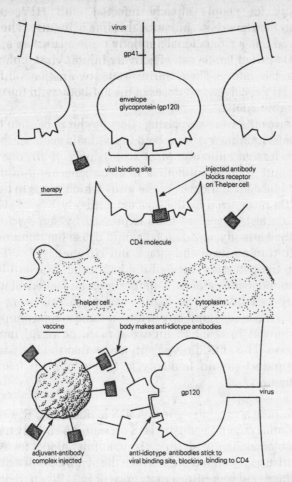

virus

gp41

envelope
glycoprotein (gp120)

viral binding site

injected antibody
blocks receptor
on T-helper cell

therapy

CD4 molecule

T-helper cell

cytoplasm

vaccine

body makes anti-idiotype antibodies

gp120

virus

adjuvant-antibody
complex injected

anti-idiotype antibodies stick to
viral binding site, blocking binding to CD4

Figure 17. One potential strategy for the treatment of HIV infection
may be to inject antibodies that recognize part of the receptor molecule on the T-helper cell. This would prevent the virus from binding to the cell. Alternatively, if such antibodies were injected as a
vaccine, in a form that stimulated the body's immune system, the
body might produce anti-idiotype antibodies that would block the
envelope protein of the virus. These, too, would prevent the virus
from attacking the T-helper cell.

189

therapy for people already infected with HIV. British researchers have been pursuing this line of inquiry. They first showed that a monoclonal antibody made against an epitope of CD4 called leu-3a can effectively inhibit viral replication in the laboratory. Then, during 1988, two patients infected with HIV received low doses of the antibody with the aim of testing its safety.

The results were surprising. Despite the poor state of the patients' immune systems, both individuals made antibodies to the foreign antibody. Most surprisingly of all, one even made anti-idiotype antibodies. In theory, these anti-idiotypes would recognize the part of the virus which binds to the site on CD4 recognized by the injected antibody.

These tests dispelled fears expressed by some scientists that the antibody, anti-leu-3a, would cause the immune system to turn on itself and attack and kill the last few T-cells left in the patients. This had not happened. The anti-leu-3a had bound to the patients' T-helper cells, and fallen off within twenty-four hours. The logical sequel to this work is to present the mouse antibody to the immune system along with an adjuvant in order to induce a more powerful immune response. The anti-idiotype antibodies that the body would then produce should, in theory, be able to 'mop up' free virus (see figure 17).

Developing a vaccine against AIDS is one thing. Evaluating a potential vaccine against AIDS presents an entirely new set of problems. First of all, there is no animal model for AIDS. Scientists can normally reproduce the symptoms of a disease in animals such as guinea pigs, mice or rats. When they want to test the efficacy of a candidate vaccine against that disease, they can inoculate the animals first with the vaccine and then, after the animals have had time to develop an immune response, with the infectious agent. They can then tell whether the vaccine protects against the disease.

In the case of HIV, humans are the only animals known to develop AIDS. Chimpanzees and gibbons do become infected when inoculated with HIV but, by late 1988, none of those infected had developed AIDS. Possibly, these primates take as long as humans do to develop AIDS – an average of eight years – so it is early days yet to conclude that they do not develop AIDS. If they do, they will provide valuable animal models for the disease.

Chimpanzees are, however, an endangered species. There are probably only about 800 captive chimps in the world available for research into AIDS. Some researchers believe that this number should meet the demand for tests of vaccines against AIDS, provided that scientists find out why the candidate vaccines that they have tried to date on chimpanzees failed to protect the animals against infection with HIV. For example, scientists in the US have vaccinated chimpanzees with vaccinia virus which had been genetically altered to manufacture the envelope protein gp160. The chimpanzees did make antibodies to HIV. The researchers then tried to infect these animals with HIV. Unfortunately, tests carried out later showed that the virus was present in all the animals.

This team, led by Shiu-Lok Hu and colleagues from the biotechnology company Oncogen, in Seattle, Washington, was cautious about drawing too many conclusions from these results, which were published in *Nature* in August 1987. The researchers suggested that the immune response may not be the same in humans as in chimpanzees. However, another group of scientists, including Jane Goodall, famous for her work on chimpanzee behaviour, wrote in *Nature* in June 1988: 'Basic research is needed to explain these failures, otherwise a long string of abortive chimpanzee trials can be anticipated.'

Attempts to find other animal models are still continuing. Ideally, scientists would like to be able to work with an animal that is small and therefore cheap and easy to keep. (As one primate researcher has said, chimps do not suffer well the indignity of captivity.) It would also be advantageous if the time from infection to onset of AIDS was short: researchers would be able to obtain their results much more quickly. In the absence of such a model, however, an alternative strategy is to work with similar viruses that cause AIDS-like diseases in other animals. For example, cats and monkeys both suffer infections caused by retroviruses, with an immune deficiency syndrome. If researchers could develop a vaccine to protect cats against infection with the feline immuno-deficiency virus, or to protect monkeys against the simian immunodeficiency virus, they might be able to apply the same techniques to make a vaccine against HIV.

The lack of an animal model explains why tests on people have taken place so early in the development of a vaccine. The tests which have taken place so far – known as Phase I tests – aim to establish only the safety of the preparations and what kind of immune response they generate. Phase I studies involve small groups of volunteers. Phase II tests are carried out on a larger group of people, including volunteers from populations which can expect to receive the vaccine if it eventually comes into general use. For Phase III studies, to test the efficacy of the candidate vaccine, the National Insti-tute of Allergy and Infectious Diseases estimates that researchers would need around 8,000 volunteers. Phase III studies would probably be randomized and placebo-con-trolled. They would take a minimum of two to three years and probably much longer, given that the period from infection to development of AIDS is, on average, about eight years.

It will be far more difficult to evaluate the efficacy of a vaccine against HIV than it has been for vaccines against many other diseases. In the absence of vaccines against dis-eases such as smallpox and whooping cough, there was little that people could do to avoid becoming infected. Scientists have traditionally tested new vaccines against such diseases on large populations of people at risk of catching the disease in question. They then establish whether the group that received the vaccine suffered fewer bouts of disease.

Such an approach is difficult with a vaccine against HIV. The risk of an adult becoming infected with HIV largely depends – in many cases, at least – on that person's behav-iour. The researchers testing such a vaccine would have an ethical obligation to educate the participants in a trial about how to avoid HIV infection. This requirement would immediately make the trial a less powerful means of determining the effectiveness of a vaccine.

Another question is, which groups should participate in trials? Should they be people at high risk or low risk of infection? In either case, would there be a risk of participants feeling a false sense of security about their risks of infection? In many countries, groups which would, several years ago, have formed ideal populations on which to test the efficacy of a vaccine, have now changed their behaviour. Transmission of the virus between homosexual men in many cities in the developed countries has virtually stopped. However, it may be possible to identify couples, whether homosexual or heterosexual, who continue to have sexual intercourse together even though one of them is infected with the virus. The uninfected partners might prove suitable people on which to test a vaccine.

It would be difficult to mount a vaccine trial among injecting drug users, too. Although the virus is spreading rapidly among people who share needles to inject drugs in developed countries, there is every sign that, given appropriate education and facilities, drug users will change their behaviour to reduce their risks. In any case, there would be problems in enrolling intravenous drug users in a vaccine trial in countries where their habit is illegal.

Considerations such as these mean that it will be very difficult to mount Phase III trials in most developed countries. Scientists trying to evaluate vaccines they have developed will have to turn to developing countries, perhaps those in Africa, for assistance. Daniel Zagury and Zaïrean colleagues have already identified which groups in Zaïre might form an appropriate testing ground for a candidate vaccine. At a conference in Africa in 1988, Zagury and his collaborators showed that there were significant differences in the spread of the virus between the cities and the countryside. More than 12 per cent of people tested in the capital of Zaïre, Kinshasa, had antibodies to the virus, compared to fewer than 5 per cent in a provincial town and fewer than 3 per cent in a rural area. When the researchers tested people who had lived in

Kinshasa for less than one year, they found only 4 per cent were positive. But more than 16 per cent of people who had lived in Kinshasa for five years or more were infected with the virus. Zagury and his colleagues concluded that young men coming from the countryside to live in Kinshasa might prove a suitable population on which to test a vaccine.

Zagury drew much criticism from some sections of the scientific community for testing his vaccine on several Zaïreans, albeit with 'the full support of the Zaïrean Ethics Committee'. To avoid tests of a doubtful ethical nature going ahead in future, particularly in developing countries, the World Health Organization is overseeing the formulation of international guidelines on the conduct of vaccine trials. The WHO hopes that these will be agreed and in place before any Phase III trials begin. The guidelines would, in particular, include guidance on what level of evidence of a vaccine's likely protective ability countries would need before agreeing to a trial of its efficacy within their borders.

Representatives from African countries have already said that initial tests to evaluate a vaccine should normally take place on volunteers from the country in which the vaccine was developed, before developing countries should consider testing it on their populations. The WHO and the Council for International Organizations of Medical Sciences have already drawn up guidelines which say that the ethical standards applied (when investigators from one country are carrying out research on subjects of another) 'should be no less exacting than they would be for research carried out within the initiating country'.

Determining such standards presents no easy task. Nicholas Christakis, of Harvard University, has summarized in the *Hastings Center Report* the ethical issues related to carrying out vaccine trials in Africa. He points out that people taking part in a Phase III trial would have to be free of HIV infection. There are several reasons for this. One is that it is impossible to evaluate the protection offered by a vaccine in people who are already infected with the infectious agent. Secondly, people infected with HIV might suffer severe side effects as a result of receiving a vaccine – particularly one based on vaccinia virus – because of the extra strain on the immune system.

To ensure that the subjects taking part in the trial were uninfected, the organizers would have to test people initially, and then test them six months later. The aim of the second test would be to eliminate people who were recently infected at the time of the first test but had not developed antibodies. In between, of course, all those volunteering to take part would have to avoid any behaviour that could put them at risk of HIV infection.

People taking part would also need to be at risk of HIV infection: if they were not, it would be impossible to evaluate the effectiveness of the vaccine. In Africa, some of the risk factors for HIV infection include having many sexual partners, having sex with prostitutes, being a prostitute or being a sexual partner of an infected person. But, Christakis says, volunteers would also have to be strongly advised to decrease the number of their sexual partners, to avoid prostitutes, and to abstain from sex with people known to be infected. It would then be necessary to make the study even larger, in order to detect a difference in the rate of infection between those who received the vaccine and those who merely followed the advice.

Another issue which must be tackled, Christakis says, is that of burdening people with the knowledge of whether they are infected with HIV. People excluded from a vaccine trial might realize that this is because they are already infected. Others might learn during the course of the trial that they had become infected. Then there is the problem that participants will become seropositive as a result of being vaccinated. (In the US, there are plans to issue such people with certificates confirming that they have taken part in a trial. It may also be possible to include some 'marker antigen' with vaccines, to which people are not normally exposed, which would make it possible to distinguish between those naturally infected and those with antibodies following vaccination.)

Christakis concludes that those people who stand to benefit from the research should be those to bear the burden of the risks of the research. 'In Central and Western Africa much of the population at large stands to gain by introduction of an effective vaccine. Yet economic constraints may well prevent even moderately extensive distribution of a beneficial vaccine in Africa, should one become available. The benefits to Africans are thus only hypothetical unless there is a financial commitment by the developed world to provide the vaccine. In this light, it would be frankly unethical to subject Africans to a disproportionate share of the research risks.'

There is also, of course, the question of informed consent. Christakis says: 'It is clear that the type of consent practised in the West, with the signing of an informed consent document containing medical terms, is inappropriate for illiterate or semi-literate peoples . . . In some cultural settings it may be extremely difficult to convey an accurate understanding of the idea of randomization or other essential scientific concepts.'

Even in many developed countries it may be difficult to explain what risks are associated with participating in a vaccine trial. So little is known about how the immune system responds to HIV that it is almost impossible to predict the consequences of the various approaches to a vaccine currently being explored. Some scientists have put forward theories that suggest that some vaccines may make matters worse, not better. Some researchers, for example, believe that the envelope protein of HIV may be directly responsible for some of the symptoms of HIV infection, particularly those affecting the nervous system.

Another theory is that, if it is true that most macrophages become infected as a result of engulfing HIV which is complexed with antibody, a vaccine which stimulates the production of antibodies would do more harm than good (see p. 173). Furthermore, what if the observations by Robert Siliciano and Ellis Reinherz and their colleagues (see p. 104) are shown to be relevant to the interactions of the virus with cells in the body, as opposed to in the test tube? Ronald Germain, of the National Institute of Allergy and Infectious Diseases, writing in the same issue of *Cell* in which Siliciano and Ellis's paper was published, suggested that candidate vaccines based on the envelope protein of the virus, gp120, must be 'examined cautiously'. The reason, he said, was that 'an individual not protected fully by such a treatment may become more susceptible to the rapid development of immunodeficiency following infection.' In other words, vaccinated individuals who nevertheless became infected with HIV might experience more severe disease as a result of their previous vaccination. There are precedents for such reactions to vaccines against viral diseases in animals. For example, in goats immunized against a viral disease that causes arthritis and encephalitis, animals later exposed to live virus suffered more severe disease.

There are still many gaps in scientists' knowledge of how HIV attacks the immune system. By the late 1980s, most attempts at a vaccine have done little more than scratch the surface of the problem. If a candidate vaccine that showed some promise of being effective were to be available tomorrow, it would still be many years before it could be properly evaluated and marketed. Even looking ahead to the day when that elusive vaccine is here, the prospects of rapidly eliminating this new disease from the world are slim. Smallpox, the greatest success story in the history of vaccination, had very different characteristics to AIDS and HIV infection. Someone with smallpox is infectious to others for a matter of a few weeks. Someone with HIV infection is probably infectious for the rest of his or her life. Smallpox produces characteristic physical signs which made it possible to identify and isolate sufferers. HIV infection does not. AIDS will be with us for long time to come.

Chapter 12

THE AFRICAN DIMENSION

When AIDS began to appear in Kinshasa, the capital of Zaïre, the first people to suffer were prostitutes in their late teens and early twenties. A little later, it was the turn of their clients, typically men in their early fifties – the 'sugar daddies', as they are commonly described. Then, babies born to infected mothers began to fall ill. Eventually, doctors became aware of AIDS in young children, infected by contaminated blood in transfusions.

The story of AIDS in Kinshasa illustrates the differences between how AIDS has spread in Africa and how it has developed in the US and Europe. In much of Africa, homosexual activity and drug abuse are uncommon. In sub-Saharan Africa, unlike the US and Europe, the human immunodeficiency virus is spreading mainly by heterosexual intercourse and from infected mothers to their children. Blood transfusions have also made an important contribution to the spread of the virus in many African countries, although facilities for screening blood are now increasingly available.

The first hints that AIDS could be present in Africa as well as the US and Europe followed the observation in 1983 that a high proportion of the cases of AIDS in Europe involved people from Africa. Doctors from Brussels reported in the *Lancet* that they had identified a group of five black Africans with AIDS. These patients, from Zaïre and Chad, had been

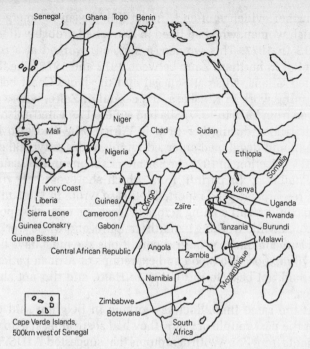

Figure 18. Most of the African countries mentioned in this chapter are shown on this map. HIV-1 is most common in central and east Africa. In west Africa, HIV-2 is more common than HIV-1.

living in Belgium for between eight months and three years. Soon after, French researchers in Paris announced twenty-nine cases of AIDS in France. These doctors found that most of their patients had travelled to the US, Haiti or equatorial Africa. Those who had gone to the US were mainly homosexual men; the rest were mainly heterosexual. The association with Africa was 'striking', the researchers said.

Another French team found AIDS in a twenty-three-year-old black woman who had left Zaïre in June 1981. She died of her infections in March 1982. The scientists warned that, along with evidence of AIDS in Haitians and haemophiliacs in the US, this case suggested that the syndrome was not restricted to homosexuals and drug abusers.

Further evidence of an 'African link' began to emerge. A Danish woman, who had lived in Zaïre, had probably died of AIDS in 1977. This woman, a surgeon, worked at a rural hospital in northern Zaïre between 1972 and 1975. She then visited Ghana, Nigeria, Senegal and the Ivory Coast before resuming work in Kinshasa, the capital of Zaïre, where she stayed from 1975 to 1977. She had suffered repeated episodes of diarrhoea during her time in Africa. She had also lost weight and developed enlarged lymph nodes, a typical sign of HIV infection. In 1977 she had attacks of pneumonia caused by *Pneumocystis carinii*, from which she eventually died. The researchers who reported her case wrote in the *Lancet*: 'She could recall coming across at least one case of Kaposi's sarcoma while working in northern Zaïre, and while working as a surgeon under primitive conditions she must have been heavily exposed to blood and excretions of African patients. She had not been to the US or to Haiti, and did not abuse drugs.'

At the same time, doctors working in Belgium said that over the past couple of years, they had seen 'at least a dozen' patients from Zaïre with symptoms that suggested AIDS. The most prominent indication of AIDS in these patients was a fungal condition called cryptococcosis. Only wealthier people in Zaïre could afford to come for treatment in Europe, these doctors pointed out, so the cases they had seen were probably the tip of the iceberg.

These doctors also described the case of a thirty-four-year-old black woman from Zaïre, who, they said, had probably had AIDS in 1977. This woman, a secretary with an airline company, had had three healthy children by her first husband. She had remarried and had three more children by her second husband. Of these three, the two eldest had already died by August 1977, when she brought the third child from her second marriage to Belgium for medical treatment. While she was in Belgium, the woman began to suffer symptoms and infections typical of AIDS. She flew back to Kinshasa, where she died in February 1978.

Later, in 1983, evidence emerged that AIDS in Africa was

not confined to Zaïre and Chad. French doctors described the case of a man from Mali who had never been to central Africa. In fact, he had lived and travelled only in Mali and France. His last visit to Mali was in 1982. He had had 'no special contact with anyone from Zaïre at home or at work'. This man had been married twice and he had four children. He did not inject drugs, he was not a haemophiliac, he had never had a blood transfusion, and, the doctors said, he was 'strictly heterosexual'. He first showed signs of illness in May 1981, eventually dying of infections typical of AIDS in June 1983. Mali is well over a thousand miles from Zaïre. AIDS, it was becoming clear, was more widely distributed in Africa than people had first thought.

Nevertheless, the link with Zaïre grew stronger. In February 1984, Nathan Clumeck and his colleagues from the Saint-Pierre University Hospital in Brussels described AIDS in twenty-two black Africans and one Greek man who had lived in Zaïre. These patients all had either opportunistic infections or Kaposi's sarcoma, or symptoms such as enlarged lymph glands, fever, loss of weight and diarrhoea. In addition, they all had immunological abnormalities typical of AIDS. None was homosexual, none used intravenous drugs and none had had a blood transfusion. Sixteen of the eighteen patients with AIDS came from Zaïre; of the remaining two, one came from Burundi, which shares a border with east rn Zaïre, and the other was from Chad in the north. By looking at the medical records of these patients, the doctors found that the earliest date of diagnosis was May 1979, in a patient from Zaïre.

Clumeck and his colleagues suggested that, because the syndrome was appearing in young to middle-aged men and women, it might be spreading by heterosexual contact. They added: 'We believe that AIDS is a new disease that is spreading in central Africa.'

Whether AIDS was a new disease or one that had been left undiagnosed for many years was difficult to determine. Perhaps, some Western researchers suggested, AIDS had always been present in Africa. Some investigations, however, supported the idea that something new was happening. Apart from cryptococcosis, other diseases seemed to be behaving oddly. The skin tumour Kaposi's sarcoma, for example, had changed from being a fairly mild condition into a fatal one.

Up to the end of the 1970s, those people who suffered from Kaposi's sarcoma in Africa were mostly older men. They developed swelling and purplish nodules on the legs and feet. Often these tumours would go away on their own but, if not, powerful drugs would do the trick. Patients often survived more than ten years with this condition.

By 1983, this description no longer held good. Anne Bayley, professor of surgery at the University Teaching Hospital in Lusaka, Zambia, said in 1983 that Kaposi's sarcoma had changed. She said, 'Whatever I do, these patients all die.'

As Kaposi's sarcoma was associated with AIDS in American homosexual men, the next step was to find out if AIDS had any connection with this new type of Kaposi's sarcoma in Africa. Bayley examined and tested patients with Kaposi's sarcoma to see whether they had antibodies to the AIDS virus. Virtually all the patients with the unusual type of Kaposi's sarcoma had antibodies to the virus. People without Kaposi's sarcoma, or with the traditional variety, were far less likely to have antibodies to the virus.

In June 1984, Bayley wrote in the *Lancet* that she could now divide her patients with Kaposi's sarcoma into two distinct groups: those with the typical disease which responded to treatment, and those with unusual symptoms who died rapidly. From 1975 to 1982, Bayley used to see up to about a dozen new patients with Kaposi's sarcoma a year, most of them with typical symptoms. By 1983, the pattern had changed. In that year, ten new patients came under Bayley's care, all of them conforming to the traditional pattern. They all got better when treated with drugs. But there was a second group of thirteen patients who appeared that year. These individuals were younger than the other group and better educated. Four of them, Bayley said, had similar jobs, suggesting an occupational or social cluster. The key characteristic, however, was that their Kaposi's sarcoma progressed rapidly

202

and did not respond well to treatment. It was, in other words, very similar to the type of tumour suffered by immunosuppressed homosexuals.

At around this time, doctors in Britain described the case of a woman from Uganda who had developed Kaposi's sarcoma. They wrote in the *Lancet*: 'To our knowledge, this is the first case of AIDS in a patient from Uganda.'

During 1983 and 1984, teams of researchers began studies to determine how widely AIDS was spreading in some African countries. One group, led by Peter Piot of the Institute of Tropical Medicine in Antwerp, in Belgium, examined patients at hospitals in Kinshasa, Zaïre. During three weeks in October 1983, they identified thirty-eight patients with AIDS.

Of these thirty-eight, the men tended to be older than the women. Men and women were affected almost equally: the male to female ratio was 1.1:1, suggesting that the disease was spread heterosexually. There was also some evidence that relatively more cases might be occurring in people with higher incomes.

Out of fifteen men questioned, thirteen said that they had had sexual intercourse with more than one woman during the year before their illness started. These men had, on average, seven sexual partners a year, though some had had as many as a hundred. Eight women patients also provided information on their sexual partners. Six of them had had more than one partner during the year before the onset of symptoms, with an average of three and a maximum of five.

Piot and his colleagues estimated that there were about seventeen cases of AIDS every year for every 100,000 people living in Kinshasa. (For comparison, about fourteen in every 100,000 single men in the US had AIDS in 1984, rising to about 340 per 100,000 in San Francisco.) If children were excluded from the population, the rate would be even higher.

These researchers also wondered about the possible origin of the disease. Although exact figures were not available, they knew that several thousand professional people had gone from Haiti to Zaïre between the early 1960s and the mid-

1970s. After talking to Haitians still living in Zaïre, the scientists concluded that most of those people had now left Zaïre and gone to live in Europe or the US. 'We were unable to identify any common factor accounting for the occurrence of AIDS in Haiti and in Zaïre almost simultaneously,' they said. They knew of only one case of AIDS among Haitians living in Zaïre – an unmarried woman in 1983. So, they concluded, they knew of no facts implicating either central Africans or Haitians as the origin of the disease.

Piot did not know when AIDS first appeared in Kinshasa. As far back as 1975, there seemed to have been some cases of weight loss, swollen lymph glands and aggressive Kaposi's sarcoma in young adults, but there was not enough information to establish these cases as AIDS. Despite the reports of probable cases of AIDS in Zaïre in 1976 and 1977, it was unlikely that African patients with AIDS seeking treatment in Europe would have gone unrecognized.

This group of researchers also noted a sharp increase in the number of cases of the fungal infection cryptococcosis in Kinshasa. Cryptococcosis is a common infection in patients with AIDS, especially those from Africa. Between the mid-1950s and late 1979, each of two hospitals in Kinshasa had, on average, one case of this infection a year. Between 1981 and early 1984, the two hospitals between them had seen more than thirty-five cases of cryptococcosis, most of them thought to have been associated with AIDS. Piot and his colleagues concluded: 'This is consistent with the emergence of the disease in large numbers simultaneously with the first cases in the USA and Haiti.'

While research continued in Zaïre, other scientists studied the situation in Kigali, the capital of Rwanda. Philippe Van de Perre and his colleagues from the Saint-Pierre University Hospital in Brussels diagnosed twenty-six patients with AIDS during a period of four weeks in late 1983. They estimated that there were eighty cases of AIDS a year for every 100,000 people living in Kigali.

Two of the twenty-six patients diagnosed were children,

both aged under two years. Of the twenty-four adults, seventeen were men and seven were women. Thirteen of the men said that they had had frequent and regular heterosexual contacts with different partners, including prostitutes in eleven cases. Three of the seven women were prostitutes; two others said that their husbands frequently went to prostitutes. So, as the researchers said, 'sexual promiscuity could be a risk factor among heterosexual patients with AIDS'. Many of the patients also had evidence of other sexually transmitted diseases such as gonorrhoea and syphilis.

Factors such as homosexuality, use of intravenous drugs and blood transfusions did not seem to figure in these cases. However, Van de Perre found that almost all the patients were middle or upper class. They concluded: 'Urban activity, a reasonable standard of living, heterosexual promiscuity and contacts with prostitutes could be risk factors for African AIDS.'

In December 1984, a local paper in Uganda published an article on an unusual illness. People in the Rakai district of Uganda, which borders the western shores of Lake Victoria, near the border with Tanzania, were wasting away and dying of diarrhoea. The local name for it was 'slim disease'. Doctors in Uganda wondered if the new illness was related to the syndrome of weight loss and diarrhoea that their colleagues in the US were reporting in homosexuals with AIDS.

The government sent a team of investigators to find out what was happening. They said that the illness did not seem to be due to outbreaks of cholera or typhoid. Then, in June, doctors in Uganda decided to mount a weekend expedition to Masaka, on the edge of the Rakai district. One of them was Anne Bayley, who was in Kampala as an external examiner for the finals exams at the medical school.

The group eventually arrived at a hospital in Masaka. Of 110 patients on the wards, the doctors could diagnose twenty-nine as having AIDS from their symptoms alone. The doctors also took blood samples. Subsequent testing showed that all these patients were positive for antibodies to the AIDS virus.

The results of this study, together with those of a survey of forty-two patients with slim disease in Kampala, most of whom also came from Masaka or the Rakai district, appeared in the *Lancet* in October 1985. When the researchers tested blood samples from the patients in Kampala who had slim disease, they found that about three-quarters of them had antibodies to the AIDS virus, too. They also tested samples of blood from 410 healthy medical staff at Mulago Hospital in Kampala; 10 per cent of them were positive.

Although the doctors described slim disease as a new syndrome, previously unreported in Uganda, it later became clear that this condition was indeed AIDS. Slim disease seemed to be a new disease in Uganda. Post mortem medical records in Uganda are good, going back to 1944. The researchers said that if slim disease had been present earlier, they would have been able to find reports of it in the records.

The first recognized cases of slim disease in Uganda occurred in a small fishing village on Lake Victoria, just north of the Tanzanian border. Villages such as this one became host to traders and smugglers in the days when road blocks in Uganda prevented goods from flowing out of the country into Tanzania. Some of the first people to suffer from slim disease were the traders. One theory is that the traders may have brought the virus back with them from Tanzania.

Bayley and her colleagues speculated about how the virus could have entered Uganda. 'The notion that the disease may have been transmitted sexually from Tanzania is interesting since it fits historically with the movements of the Tanzanian army in 1980 and the subsequent movements of the Tanzanian traders. Of the fifteen traders tested for evidence of . . . antibodies, ten were positive. These traders admitted to both heterosexual and homosexual casual contacts. Tanzanian soldiers entering Uganda since 1980 have had frequent heterosexual contact with the local population.' But the puzzle remained. 'If the virus did come from Tanzania, where did Tanzania get it from?'

By 1985, many new tests for antibodies to HIV had become

available to researchers who wanted to study the extent of infection in Africa. Teams of scientists mounted expeditions to remote areas to find out how far the virus had spread. Others carried out tests on samples of blood serum that had been taken years before and stored frozen. They wanted to find out exactly when the virus had appeared in Africa. The figures that began to appear at first sight suggested, rather surprisingly, that the epidemic was older and more extensive than anyone had first thought.

For example, Carl Saxinger of the National Cancer Institute in the US, and his colleagues, found, in a study that would later be discredited, that over 60 per cent of healthy children in the West Nile district of Uganda had, in the early 1970s, had antibodies to the AIDS virus. Saxinger and his co-workers wrote in *Science*, '. . . it is likely that residents of the West Nile region of Uganda have been and continue to be exposed to the virus at a very early age'. They also suggested: 'It is possible that AIDS existed in African populations without being recognized as a separate disease entity. The virus may have originated in Africa in the past and exposure to the virus may be much more common than AIDS itself in some populations.'

Robert Biggar, also of the National Cancer Institute, published the results of several studies carried out around 1984. In a remote part of eastern Zaïre, for example, he found that over 12 per cent of 250 Zaïrean hospital outpatients had 'clearly positive' results to tests for antibodies to the virus. According to Biggar, another 12 per cent had 'borderline' results. Yet none of these patients had symptoms suggesting AIDS. Furthermore, no case of AIDS had ever been diagnosed at the hospital where these tests were carried out.

Biggar, together with American and Kenyan collaborators, also tested samples of blood taken from people all over Kenya during 1980 and 1984. Overall, about one in five of almost seven hundred people tested seemed to have antibodies to the virus, with another 24 per cent of those tested having 'borderline' reactions. Antibodies to the virus seemed to be more common in people from some parts of Kenya rather than others. For example, half of the ninety-nine people tested from the remote Turkana district had positive results.

There were warning signs that something might be wrong with these results. In the Kenyan study, the researchers mentioned that they knew of only three cases of AIDS in Kenya, all diagnosed in Nairobi. As the quality of medical care in Kenya was quite good, it seemed odd that cases of AIDS were not appearing at a rate which would reflect the number of people in the population apparently infected with the virus.

Biggar and his colleagues speculated on why this should be the case. Perhaps the manifestations of AIDS in Africa were different to those in the US and Europe. Perhaps the course of infection was different in Africa. If people became infected as children, maybe the virus did not kill them; if it did, perhaps the people with antibodies were those who had survived infection. There was a third theory: perhaps infection alone did not cause abnormalities of the immune system. Some other factor which caused AIDS to develop in infected people in the US and Europe may have been missing in Africa. Finally, Biggar suggested, maybe the virus was just less virulent in Africa.

In fact, the cause of these odd results was probably that blood serum from Africans reacted with the proteins present in the tests, even though these people had no antibodies to the AIDS virus. In other words, they were false positives.

Biggar revised his opinions. In early 1986, he wrote that knowledge of the spread of AIDS in Africa had been hampered by 'lack of data and perhaps misleading preliminary laboratory results'. When he tested for the second time forty-six healthy people from Zaïre and Kenya whom he had originally believed to be infected with the virus, he found only two that had results typical of true positives. Surveys in Africa, he said, had probably greatly overestimated the extent of the spread of HIV. Similarly, tests on repeatedly frozen and thawed blood samples taken from African children more than a decade ago – as in Saxinger's study – had probably also resulted in overestimates.

Biggar reviewed the evidence that AIDS was, in fact, a

new disease in Africa. 'In my conversations with clinicians practising in tropical Africa during the 1960s and 1970s, they have stated strongly that if AIDS had existed as anything other than rare, sporadic cases, it would have been recognized . . .' Similarly, cases of Africans seeking medical advice in Europe for diseases associated with AIDS only began to appear since 1980. Furthermore, the fact that AIDS is spreading in Africa 'strengthens the probability that it is a new disease'. And, Biggar added, 'There is no conclusive evidence that the AIDS virus originated in Africa, since the epidemic seemed to start at approximately the same time as in America and Europe.'

The search for the virus throughout Africa continued. By 1985, there had been only a handful of reports of AIDS in west Africa. An odd feature of some of these cases was that, although these people had symptoms typical of AIDS, when doctors tested their blood for antibodies against HIV, the results were negative. Scientists from Lisbon, in Portugal, and from Paris, including Luc Montagnier, decided to take a closer look at two such patients from west Africa.

One of these individuals was a man from Guinea-Bissau, who began to suffer symptoms of diarrhoea and loss of weight, as well as swollen lymph glands, in 1983. He also had infections typical of AIDS. The second patient was born in and lived in the Cape Verde islands, 500 kilometres off the coast of Senegal. He had first developed symptoms in January 1982; doctors in France diagnosed AIDS in June 1983. Tests for antibodies to HIV in both these patients were repeatedly negative.

The scientists managed to isolate viruses from both men. Powerful photographs of infected cells, taken using an electron microscope, showed a virus with an unusual appearance: instead of the viral membrane appearing relatively smooth, it was covered with spikes. The virus was different to the original HIV, and was later called HIV-2.

Later, many of the same researchers reported another thirty cases of AIDS caused by HIV-2, almost all of them in people from west Africa. Many of these people came from Guinea-Bissau, and two came from Cape Verde. One was an eleven-year-old boy from Angola who had lived in Cape Verde for several years. Finally, there was a forty-year-old Portuguese man who had lived for eight years in Zaïre and who said he had never stayed in west Africa. From the characteristics of these patients, it seemed that HIV-2, like HIV-1, was transmitted mainly by heterosexual contact.

A new epidemic of AIDS could be about to occur in west Africa, the scientists warned, this time caused by HIV-2. This virus was already spreading in west Africa. A survey of 275 people working at the Ministry of Health in Guinea-Bissau took place in 1986 and 1987. Almost one in five of the women were positive for HIV-2, but fewer than one in fifty had antibodies to HIV-1. Among the men, over one in ten had antibodies to HIV-2 but none had signs of infection with HIV-1. In fifty-four healthy blood donors in Guinea-Bissau, only a couple were positive for HIV-1, while more than one in four had antibodies to HIV-2. The only known risk factor for those who were infected with either virus was contact with female prostitutes.

Both HIV-1 and HIV-2 seemed to have been present in the population in Guinea-Bissau for some time. The researchers tested 300 samples of blood taken and stored in 1980. In three (1 per cent) they found antibodies to HIV-1; a further six (2 per cent) were positive for HIV-2.

Surveys in other west African countries, such as Guinea Conakry, Ivory Coast and Benin have generally shown low levels of infection with HIV-1 and HIV-2 of the order of 1 or 2 per cent or less in the general population, although some surveys have found levels in pregnant women, for example, as high as 6 per cent. As in central Africa, prostitutes seem to be a group at high risk of infection with HIV. In Ivory Coast, between 16 per cent and 65 per cent of prostitutes tested had antibodies to either HIV-1 or HIV-2.

In central Africa, the ratio of infected men to infected women is usually close to 1:1. In Ghana in 1986, however, the ratio was almost 12:1. By 1987, the ratio had dropped to just over 6:1, which suggested to researchers that the infection was still spreading among susceptible people.

Many researchers believe that AIDS caused by HIV-2 has a much longer incubation period than that caused by HIV-1. For example, there is the case of a Portuguese man and his wife who were diagnosed as having AIDS due to HIV-2 infection. The man had done his military service in Guinea-Bissau between 1966 and 1969. Doctors investigating the couple suggested that AIDS may have taken between sixteen and nineteen years to develop in the man and eleven years in his wife. Another case, although the evidence for a long incubation period is less clear, occurred in a Portuguese man who died of AIDS in 1980. Between 1968 and 1974 he had lived and worked in Angola, both in the navy and as a truck driver from Angola to Mozambique. He first developed signs typical of HIV infection in February 1977, and went on to suffer infections typical of AIDS. Scientists tested a sample of his blood which they had stored in 1979, for antibodies to both HIV -1 and HIV-2. Antibodies to the envelope of HIV-2 were present.

Researchers who looked at the pattern of the first recognized cases of HIV-2 infection were struck by a common characteristic. Many of the infected people were either Portuguese, or from African countries linked by the former Portuguese trading routes. By 1987, cases of infection with HIV-2 had been reported in several African countries, including Cape Verde, Ghana, Guinea-Bissau, Guinea Conakry, Ivory Coast, Mali, Niger, Mozambique and Senegal. Mali and Niger, although not on the coast, are connected to it by the Niger river. Some cases have also had connections with Angola, another former Portuguese colony.

Some scientists believe that this pattern may provide a clue to the origin and subsequent spread of HIV-2. In previous centuries, the Portuguese ruled the seas. Cape Verde, for example, was an obligatory stop for ships going to South America. Researchers have suggested looking for HIV-2 in other places that the Portuguese visited, such as Goa (in India), Brazil and Cuba. By 1987, there had already been one report that HIV-2 was present in Brazil. (This virus, although it is much less common in developed countries than HIV-1, is also spreading to North America and Europe. In 1988, there were isolated reports of its presence in both the US and some European countries.)

HIV-1, by the mid-1980s, was spreading rapidly in Central and East Africa. Social and economic factors assisted the virus in its stealthy movement through the continent. The wars and political upheavals that many African countries have suffered in the past few decades have no doubt played their part in disseminating AIDS. Large movements of people – armies, refugees or those seeking jobs, for example – probably helped to widen the epidemic. In other places, it may have taken just a few highly sexually active people to sow the virus in a previously unaffected population. Geographic factors, such as lakes, mountains and rift valleys, have undoubtedly stood in the way of the virus. And, as one doctor said: 'Sexual isolation may have a lot to do with the quality of the roads.'

The virus has certainly been spreading along trade routes within Africa. The port of Mombasa is the point of entry for many goods destined for Kenya, Uganda, south Sudan, north-west Zaïre, Rwanda, Burundi and part of Tanzania. A main road leads from Mombasa, passing through Nairobi, around the top of Lake Victoria, and down through south-western Uganda (see figure 19). It skirts the northern border of Rwanda and carries on into Zaïre, eventually ending up at Kinshasa on the Congo river. Between Kampala and the Ugandan border with Zaïre, the road passes through a small town called Lyantonde.

Lyantonde is one of several small towns along the road that exist to cater for the needs of the truck drivers who transport goods to and from the ports. With a population of about four or five thousand people, it has about thirty bars and lodges. At dusk, lorries and trailers line the main street. In Lyantonde, the lorry drivers and their mates, called 'turn boys', can find a meal, beer and women.

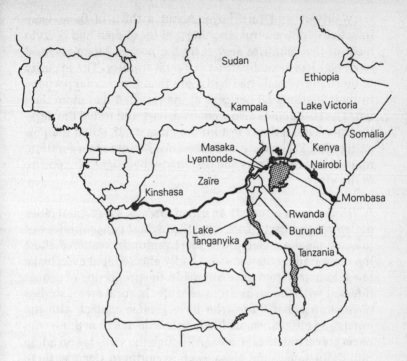

Figure 19. The road that runs between Mombasa on the east coast and Kinshasa in the west. Some of the towns and villages that are mentioned in this chapter are also shown.

Many of the women work as 'bar girls'. They are essentially prostitutes working in bars, where they get food and a uniform. Most of them are aged between about sixteen and twenty-five and come from the surrounding countryside. They usually have at least one sexual partner a day, receiving in return, if not money, goods such as paraffin or sugar.

Between 1986 and 1987, researchers in Uganda tested almost two hundred of the bar girls for antibodies to HIV. About two-thirds of them were positive. For comparison, the researchers also tested mothers and their children attending an immunization clinic. About 17 per cent of these women were infected, as well as just over 1 per cent of the children.

The next group to have blood tests comprised seventy-four

lorry drivers and turn boys. About a third of them were infected with the virus, too. Most of these men had been to most of the countries served by the port of Mombasa, and most had had sexual partners in each country. The majority of these individuals had had more than fifty sexual partners in their lifetime: 80 per cent of the rest had had more than ten. The researchers also went back later and tested the negative men with a direct test for the virus itself, rather than for antibodies. When they took these results into consideration, up to half of the drivers and their mates had signs of exposure to the virus.

AIDS in Africa is mainly an urban disease. The capital cities of Central and East Africa have the highest concentrations of infected people. Small towns like Lyantonde, scattered along the main trade routes, are also badly affected, but even just a few kilometres from the main roads, the proportion of people infected with the virus drops sharply. In rural areas, studies have shown that those who have greater contact with the towns and cities are more likely to be infected than those who never travel outside the area. Although the virus is spreading rapidly in some rural areas, such as northern Uganda, there are often special factors to account for this atypical pattern. Social disruption caused by armies and civil wars, for example, may be to blame.

One of the problems that scientists face in trying to work out the overall picture of AIDS and HIV infection in Africa is that information is very patchy. This unevenness sometimes reflects the fact that little research has been done; or it may indicate that governments are refusing to release the results, fearful of publicity that may, for example, affect their tourist trade. In 1988, Zimbabwe declared that in order to classify someone as having AIDS, it would be necessary to confirm that HIV infection was present by carrying out a second test – the sensitive Western blot test. This test, which is relatively expensive for a developing country with a limited budget for health care, is not available throughout most of Zimbabwe. Unless Zimbabwe changes its rules, the future chances of this country reporting cases of AIDS at a level which reflects the true incidence of the disease within its borders seem rather slim.

Zimbabwe began to clamp down on information about AIDS at around the time that some other African countries began to speak more freely. At the third international conference on AIDS in Africa, held in Arusha, Tanzania, in September 1988, there was a new atmosphere of frank and open discussion. Speakers and delegates were in many cases able to present and discuss the latest data on the spread of the virus without fears that governments would try to suppress disturbing figures. Tanzanian researchers, for example, presented the results of several important studies. In the Kagera region in the north of the country, to the west of Lake Victoria, researchers selected a random sample of people and tested them for antibodies to HIV. Out of almost 2,500 adults, almost 12 per cent were infected with the virus. In urban areas, about one in three adults were infected, compared with fewer than one in a hundred in a rural area. More than 40 per cent of urban adults aged twenty-five to thirty-four years old were infected with the virus.

Figures from the Mwanza region of Tanzania, south of Lake Victoria, also showed a worrying level of infection. There, almost one in twenty blood donors and more than one in twenty pregnant women were infected with the virus. In Dar es Salaam, the capital of Tanzania, a survey in 1988 of more than 200 barmaids showed that almost 40 per cent were infected, compared to 29 per cent in 1986. During the conference, the local Tanzanian newspaper, the *Daily News*, also reported that 'in some countries in Central and East Africa, an average of 18 per cent of healthy blood donors and pregnant mothers are infected'. According to local journalists, such openness would have been unthinkable even a year before.

By the late 1980s, however, many African countries were still keeping their data to themselves. Some were not publishing results showing the extent of the virus's spread at all. Others did release the information – after a fashion. In 1988, Rwanda, for example, published the results of a national survey to detect HIV infection in a government publication obtainable only from the Ministry of Health in Rwanda. This survey showed that in Kigali, the capital, one in five people tested had antibodies to the virus. One in ten of those tested who lived in small towns were positive, but fewer than two in a hundred people in rural areas were infected.

By 1988, every sub-Saharan country in Africa was at least reporting cases of AIDS to the WHO. Late that year, out of 111,000 cases reported by 140 countries around the world, almost 15,000 were from Africa. But it was clear that the numbers of cases reported bore little relation to the numbers of people who had the disease. Take Zaïre as an example. In June 1987, it had reported 335 cases of AIDS. No further report had reached the WHO by September 1988. At the conference in Arusha, James Chin, of the WHO, pointed out that Jonathan Mann, director of the WHO's Global Programme on AIDS, had personally seen more than 335 cases of AIDS when he worked for several years in Zaïre.

Chin, together with a researcher called Steve Lwanga, told the conference that probably only a tenth of the cases of AIDS that have occurred since the epidemic began have been reported to the WHO. The two scientists presented a statistical model on which they had based this statement. The model suggested that a hypothetical East African country with a population of 16.1 million would have had more than 24,000 cases of AIDS between the notional start of the epidemic, in 1980, and the end of 1987. There are about a dozen countries in Central and East Africa with a similar pattern of HIV infection, Chin said. Yet by September 1988, no sub-Saharan country in Africa had reported more than 5,000 cases of AIDS to the WHO.

Chin and Lwanga developed their model in order to help countries plan for the future health needs of their populations. In developed countries, projections of the numbers of cases of AIDS have been based largely on the numbers of cases of AIDS reported to date. In many developing countries, however, the reported number of cases is unreliable. So Chin and Lwanga worked out a way of predicting the future numbers of AIDS cases from data on the spread of the virus in different sections of the population.

The two scientists took 1980 as the year when the virus first began to spread widely in the hypothetical country. Next, they had to estimate the prevalence of the virus in the country at a specific time – the current year, for example – using the available data on the spread of the virus. People found to be infected in any one year will not all have caught their infection during that year. So Chin and Lwanga distributed the number of infections back through the previous few years to 1980. Then, using information on the rates at which infected people go on to develop AIDS, they would be able to calculate the expected number of cases of AIDS over the next few years. For example, American research suggests that 15 to 20 per cent of people develop AIDS within five years of infection, 50 per cent within ten years and 15 per cent within fifteen years.

The final ingredient of the model is an estimate of what the future incidence of HIV infection might be. (The incidence of an infection is the number of new infections in a defined group during a defined period of time.) This figure is difficult to estimate, but it does not greatly affect the predicted number of cases of AIDS during the following five years because most of these cases will be in people already infected with the virus.

Chin and Lwanga applied their model to a hypothetical East African country. They gave the country a population of 16.1 million. The structure of the population was typical. Over 40 per cent of people living in towns and cities were under fifteen years old; in the countryside, this figure was 50 per cent. And 15 per cent of the total population lived in urban areas

The next step was to take the available data on the spread of HIV in different sectors of the populations of Central and East African countries and fit these figures to the population of the hypothetical country. The researchers told the conference that surveys in some urban areas during 1986 had shown that up to 25 per cent of people aged twenty to forty years were infected with HIV. One in ten children under the age of five was also infected, as a result of transmission during pregnancy or childbirth from infected mothers. On the other hand, children aged five to fourteen years old were largely uninfected.

These figures mean that, in the hypothetical country in 1986, 12 per cent of people in urban areas were infected. In the countryside, fewer than 1 per cent were infected. Throughout the entire population, the proportion infected in 1986 would have stood at 2.6 per cent, or 416,000 people.

The WHO scientists then used the model to predict what might happen in the future. Lwanga told the conference that even if all new infection was to cease by the end of 1988, there would still be 608,000 HIV-infected people in the hypothetical country by the end of 1991. By that time, the country would have experienced 44,500 new cases of AIDS, and its total number of cases since the notional start of the epidemic would be about 87,000.

Another scenario is that which would occur if the number of new cases of HIV infection continued to grow steadily at a rate of 25 per cent a year from 1986 onwards. In this case, by 1991, there would be nearly 1.8 million HIV-positive people in the hypothetical country, which would, by that time, have experienced 126,000 cases of AIDS since the beginning of the epidemic.

Chin and Lwanga also looked at what might happen if the rate of increase of HIV infection was greatest in the early and mid-1980s and may be beginning to slow down in some areas. In this event, there would be 1.05 million HIV-positive people by 1991, and 107,500 cases of AIDS since the start of the epidemic.

The model assumes that once infected people develop AIDS, they survive only eighteen months. It also applies to HIV infection and AIDS in adults only, because the course of the disease is different in infants infected by their mothers. Furthermore, the model ignores the fact that people infected with HIV might die of unrelated causes. The effect of this omission would be to overestimate slightly the numbers of

218

HIV-infected people and cases of AIDS. Chin and Lwanga emphasized that it would be important to adjust the model as fresh data became available, and regularly re-examine the assumptions on which it was based. Nevertheless, Lwanga concluded: 'This is better than planning in a total void.'

Chin went on to tell the conference that, on the basis of this model, the WHO believed that many African countries had, by 1988, reported only about a tenth of the number of cases of AIDS that had occurred since the epidemic began. Although some members of the audience were surprised at the size of the shortfall in the official figures, Chin told delegates: 'AIDS programme managers of some countries have come up with similar figures for what they feel might be out there.'

Later, Chin explained that the factor of ten applied only to cases that had occurred since the epidemic began. Before 1985, both recognition of the disease and acceptance of its existence had been a problem in some countries. Although formal reporting began in 1986 in most countries, by the late 1980s, surveillance was still incomplete and inaccurate. Many doctors are confused about the diagnosis of AIDS and do not know whether they need a laboratory test in order to make the diagnosis. (They do not. The WHO has issued guidelines to help doctors diagnose AIDS on the basis of the patient's symptoms alone.) Another factor which makes it difficult for some countries to report all cases is that some people with AIDS never see a doctor at all. And the primary cause of death in some of those who do reach medical attention may be infections such as tuberculosis (a common opportunistic infection associated with AIDS in Africa); such deaths may be recorded as due to tuberculosis rather than to AIDS.

By 1988, some countries in East and Central Africa were getting to grips with the problem of accurate reporting. Uganda, for example, set up a surveillance system for AIDS. By May 1988, this country had reported almost 5,000 cases of AIDS – more than any other country in sub-Saharan Africa. But because of the vagaries of reporting, this does not necessarily mean that Uganda has the most cases. James Chin of

WHO estimated in late 1988 that current reports of numbers of cases of AIDS probably represent a quarter or a third of the true number, rather than a tenth.

One aspect of AIDS in Africa that has puzzled researchers for a long time is why the virus has already spread so widely among heterosexuals in parts of that continent. By contrast, in many developed countries, such as those in North America and Western Europe, the spread of the virus among heterosexuals has, at least so far, been relatively limited (see Chapter 13). In the mid-1980s, many theories were put forward to explain this difference. These theories included sweeping generalizations about sexual behaviour 'in Africa'. For example, there was much talk of 'promiscuity'. Rumours abounded, with little evidence to support them, that anal intercourse was common between men and women in Africa, either to preserve virginity or as a method of contraception. Such theories probably arose from a reluctance to admit that the virus can spread by conventional heterosexual intercourse.

Sexual behaviour does, of course, greatly influence the spread of AIDS. In any society, the more sexual partners a person has, the more likely it is that he or she will encounter someone with a sexually transmitted disease. One researcher succinctly summed up the range of human sexual behaviour. First, he said, there are the 'inactives'. Then, there are those who are more-or-less monogamous. Next come the 'fast trackers', followed finally by the professionals. These categories probably apply to all societies; what differs, according to time, place and history, is the proportion of people in each category. Societies that have undergone great economic and political upheaval are likely to have different proportions of fast trackers and professionals than societies that have remained relatively stable.

In Africa, even though the majority of people still live in the countryside, there has been a tremendous influx of people to the towns and cities in the past couple of decades. Many men go to the cities to find work, leaving their families at home. On their own in the cities, they may be 'predisposed to casual sexual behaviour', as one Ugandan researcher put it.

Many researchers believe that the urban lifestyle is to blame for the rapid spread of the virus. At the second international conference on AIDS in Africa, held in Naples in October 1987, African delegates were quick to protest when one European researcher implied that 'promiscuity' could be an explanation for the African epidemic. Nathan Clumeck, of St Peter's Hospital in Brussels, Belgium, told the meeting that promiscuity was difficult to define. Nevertheless, he added, 'we can assume' that the number of partners in some groups in Africa may be higher than in the West.

Gottlieb Monekosso, director of the WHO's regional office for Africa, later told journalists: 'There is no way you can practise promiscuity in an African village.' Africans, he added, are no more or less promiscuous than anybody else, given the same social freedom. He saw AIDS as an urban problem, among people whose lifestyle was not very different from that of young Westerners. People who could travel, with access to hotels and 'all the freedom you have when you are free to do what you care to do' were most at risk.

The issue of promiscuity was still bubbling away at the third conference on AIDS in Africa, one year later. Samuel Okware, head of the Ugandan AIDS control programme, said that he had studied the sexual behaviour of a group of people. He found that the average number of partners over a period of five years was 5.6. The audience applauded when he said: 'I think that one sexual partner per year is the minimum required to meet the physiological needs of any African. This is irrefutable evidence that we are not really promiscuous.'

Unfortunately, one partner a year every year for five years could be enough to put someone at high risk of becoming infected with HIV in areas where one in three or one in four young adults is infected with the virus. Nevertheless, sexual behaviour cannot be the sole explanation for the different pattern of the epidemic in Africa. Studies of couples in which one partner is infected with the virus have produced conflict-

221

ing results between Africa and the US. In Africa, some studies have shown that the virus has passed to the other partner in 70 per cent of cases. In the US and Europe, the figure is frequently much lower, at around 20 or 25 per cent. Studies in Europe and the US have frequently failed to find any correlation between the number of occasions that sexual intercourse took place and transmission to the previously uninfected partner.

Research presented at Arusha provided clues to the other factors which may influence the spread of the virus. Francis Plummer, of the University of Nairobi, in Kenya, reported that men with genital ulcer disease – a general term for different kinds of ulcers, including chancroid and those caused by syphilis and herpes – were far more likely to be infected with HIV than those without. Uncircumcised men were also at higher risk of HIV infection than circumcised men.

Plummer had also earlier published, in the *New England Journal of Medicine*, the results of a study which found no correlation between the number of sexual partners a man had during his lifetime and his risk of being infected with HIV. Out of thirty-eight men infected with HIV, just over half had had between ten and fifty sexual partners during their lifetime, compared to just under half of 302 men who were not infected with HIV. The difference was not statistically significant.

Plummer and his colleagues had set out to identify risk factors for the transmission of HIV. They had already tested a thousand prostitutes in one district of Nairobi, and found that 85 per cent were infected with the virus. Next, they concentrated on men attending a clinic for sexually transmitted diseases in Nairobi who said they had visited prostitutes in that area. Out of 429 men recruited to the study, 370 were initially free of the virus. But by the end of one year, 16 per cent of this group – slightly more than one in six – had developed antibodies to HIV.

Almost half of the men who became infected had an intact foreskin as well as genital ulcer disease. By contrast, only very few of those who were circumcised and had no history of genital ulcer disease became infected with HIV. When Plummer and his colleagues tried to estimate the risk of infection following a single contact with a prostitute, they concluded that men who were uncircumcised were eight times more likely to become infected with HIV. (These men did not have genital ulcer disease.)

The foreskin may act as a physical trap for the virus, Plummer said. As mild inflammation under the foreskin is quite common, this could provide a portal of entry for HIV. Plummer also pointed out that the areas where the HIV epidemic is most severe fit well with the geographic pattern of male circumcision in Africa. West Africa, where spread has been less rapid, is 'pretty solidly circumcised', he said. But circumcision is less common in countries such as Uganda, Burundi and Rwanda.

In their article in the *New England Journal of Medicine*, Plummer and his colleagues noted that no previously published studies had shown a link between lack of circumcision and HIV infection. But this may have been overlooked as a risk factor for homosexuals, they suggested, because 85 per cent of American white men are circumcised.

At Arusha, Plummer told journalists that he would recommend circumcision, providing there were no ethnic objections to it. But he added: 'The central fact of the epidemiology of HIV is that there is a subgroup of people who are very sexually active who maintain this disease in the population – essentially prostitutes and their clients.' If it were possible to control the disease in those groups, it would be possible to control transmission, Plummer said. The way to do this would be by promoting the use of condoms and reducing the number of cases of sexually transmitted diseases.

It is sometimes difficult to translate the figures of predicted cases of AIDS into human suffering. AIDS strikes people down during their most economically productive years. Particularly in those parts of Africa where the epidemic is most severe, the effects on all levels of society will be, if they are not already, immense. In some regions of Uganda, for example, virtually every family has lost someone from AIDS. By the early 1990s, that statement will apply to a much larger area (including, most probably, parts of Latin America). The ramifications of AIDS will spread far and wide.

At the level of the family, there are children who have lost their parents. Their upbringing will be left to their grandparents – who will, in turn, have lost the only social security they ever had, their sons or daughters. The impact on societies in general will depend largely on which sectors of the population are most widely infected. Many questions remain unanswered. In places where many agricultural workers are infected, will food production suffer? What will happen in countries where one in three soldiers in the army is infected? What about societies where the most severely afflicted are those who are highly educated and those whose technical and administrative skills are sorely needed? AIDS, as Jonathan Mann, director of the WHO's Global Programme on AIDS, has often said, threatens the political and economic stability of many nations.

The cost of HIV infection and AIDS in Africa is difficult to estimate. There is the direct cost of treating people with AIDS. There is also the indirect cost, which officials of the World Bank have defined as the value of the healthy years of life AIDS steals from society. The World Bank estimates that in a country such as Tanzania, for example, the direct cost per person could range from $104 to $631, depending on whether patients choose to seek the best available modern care, or remain in their village, cared for by relatives. But these figures do not take into account the costs of the health care forgone by patients crowded out of the health care system by people with AIDS.

The World Bank has also calculated how many healthy years of life would be saved by preventing one case of HIV infection. When this calculation takes into account the productivity of the healthy years of life saved, it turns out that every case of HIV infection prevented saves six to seven years of life, more than would be saved by preventing many other diseases. The bank estimates that the cost of the healthy, productive years lost through HIV infection – the indirect cost – ranges from almost $2,500 to just over $5,000 per person in Tanzania.

It is undeniable that many thousands of people will die from AIDS in Africa over the next couple of decades. However, because the populations of many African countries are growing very rapidly, AIDS may not cause populations to fall. A British researcher, Roy Anderson, has developed a model to try to determine what impact AIDS will have on the populations of African countries. According to his calculations, AIDS may or may not turn the rate of population growth from positive to negative. It is more likely to turn rates of growth negative if a high proportion of people infected with HIV develop AIDS and die, and if a high proportion of babies born to infected women are also infected and die. Anderson also calculates that if AIDS does reverse the trend of population growth, it will take a long time for the population to begin to decline after the introduction of HIV – perhaps several decades. But he warns that his predictions should be treated with caution, because so little is known about factors such as the rates at which people change their sexual partners, how long HIV infection and AIDS take to incubate in developing countries, and the likelihood of an infected person passing the virus on to others, and of an infected woman infecting her child.

Many African countries still take the view that AIDS is not their number one problem. At the second international conference on AIDS in Africa, held in Naples in October 1987, Gottlieb Monekosso, director of the WHO's regional office for Africa in Brazzaville, said that AIDS does not represent the same threat that it does in Europe or the US. AIDS, he said, probably ranks only tenth or lower on a list of serious tropical diseases. Malaria, measles, diarrhoeal illnesses, tuberculosis, cholera, meningitis, yellow fever and various cancers all kill more people than AIDS does.

In October 1988, at the third conference on AIDS in Africa, held in Arusha, many delegates repeated the message that diseases such as malaria must maintain their claim to funding and resources. How can African countries where the annual health budget per person may be as low as $1 cope with so many competing demands on their health services? To help countries meet the extra demands imposed by AIDS, the WHO set up its Global Programme on AIDS in February 1987. The WHO estimated in 1988 that the programme would need funds of $66.2m in the same year, more than three-quarters of which would go to support national AIDS programmes.

The WHO raises money for national programmes by holding meetings between governments of countries seeking assistance and those of donor nations, as well as international aid agencies. By August 1988, fourteen African countries had established national AIDS programmes in conjunction with the WHO, with pledged funding totalling more than $54m. Countries will use the money to develop education and information programmes to help to limit the spread of HIV, as well as to train medical staff and set up surveys to study the progress of the epidemic. Other aspects of the control programmes include ensuring that medical instruments such as syringes are properly sterilized, and that donated blood is screened for antibodies to the virus.

In the view of some cynics, the West gives money for AIDS simply because, unlike many tropical diseases present in Africa, AIDS poses a threat to travellers from developed countries: this is why so much attention has been focused on cleansing the blood supply in Africa. It has also been said that AIDS cannot be controlled until it is controlled in all countries. In the light of this comment, it is interesting to ponder what will happen if scientists manage to develop a vaccine effective against HIV. Sadly, effective vaccines against many infectious diseases have failed to lift the burden of these diseases from people in many developing countries. It is a chastening thought that even though there is an effective vaccine against tetanus, for example, this disease still kills 80,000 children a year. Measles, another disease against which many children in the developed world are routinely vaccinated, kills a child somewhere in the world every fifteen seconds: two million every year. Every year, around two million children under the age of five suffer from tuberculosis (another disease for which a vaccine is available), at least 30,000 of whom will die as a result of the infection. No wonder some African countries question the eagerness to pour money into controlling AIDS, when so many other treatable or preventable diseases cause so much illness and so many deaths among their citizens.

Despite the multitude of demands on their resources, however, many African countries are now tackling the threat of AIDS with a new vigour. Uganda, for example, has one of the best programmes in Africa to educate people about AIDS. There is even some evidence that the message is getting through: some reports from Uganda suggest that the level of sexually transmitted diseases in some urban areas has dropped sharply.

Lars Kallings, the eminent Swedish scientist, summing up after the Arusha conference on AIDS in Africa, questioned why there was not a greater sense of urgency about the problem. Perhaps, he said, it was because people feel helpless in the face of the epidemic. 'In only a couple of years,' he said, 'I'm afraid that there will be a frightening body count.' There were signs, he added, that the body count can change behaviour. There was also reason for a great deal of hope. In most African countries, about 50 per cent of the population are aged under fifteen. And children under fifteen, apart from those infected at birth, are largely spared from infection with HIV.

Conjecture about where the AIDS virus came from — there was only one virus in those days — has abounded ever since doctors first identified the existence of the epidemic. Unfortunately, some of the early attempts to pinpoint the origin of AIDS were confused because of a laboratory mix-up. The researchers involved were Max Essex and Phyllis Kanki, from the Harvard School of Public Health in Boston. They said they had found a link between human immunodeficiency viruses and similar viruses that infect monkeys. For nearly two years, the world believed that Essex and Kanki had discovered a 'missing link' suggesting that AIDS had originated in Africa. They suggested that the human virus had evolved from a similar virus that infects African green monkeys. Unfortunately, this idea was based on inaccurate data.

Essex said that the new virus that he 'discovered' in 1986 came from blood samples taken from Senegalese prostitutes. He called the virus HTLV-4, in the style of Robert Gallo's HTLV-3. Essex's announcement closely followed Luc Montagnier's disclosure to the press that he had also found a new virus. This virus, also found in West Africans, eventually became known as HIV-2. (The coincidental timing of the two announcements was evidently the result of personal rivalry between the two sets of researchers: in science, being first with a discovery is important.)

On superficial examination, HTLV-4 bore a close similarity to another retrovirus which Essex had announced the discovery of several months earlier, back in 1985. This virus, Essex claimed, had been isolated from African green monkeys, and he called it STLV-3 (the name stands for simian T-lymphotrophic virus). The similarity between the two viruses suggested that they were related. People speculated that the ancestor of the African green monkey virus had somehow 'jumped' from monkeys to humans, perhaps a long time ago.

During 1987, however, some researchers began to suspect that Essex and Kanki had made a mistake. When they began to look at the genetic structure of HTLV-4, they found that it was closely similar to a virus that another team of researchers, from the New England Regional Primate Research Center in Massachusetts, had found in macaque monkeys.

Many researchers suspected that Essex had not, in fact, isolated a human virus, but that his sample had become contaminated with the virus already isolated from macaques. The New England researchers had, after all, sent him samples of this virus. Such contamination is not unheard of and researchers normally take careful steps to prevent it.

To try to confirm the true identity of HTLV-4, one AIDS

researcher, Abraham Karpas, from the University of Cambridge in England, even wrote to the journal *Nature* in 1987 asking the editor to publish a letter saying that HTLV-4 was one and the same as the macaque virus. The journal, however, said that it was inappropriate to publish such a letter. Meanwhile, even informed AIDS researchers continued to believe in the validity of HTLV-4.

Eventually, however, scientists from the New England primate centre published the full genetic sequences of both their macaque virus and the two viruses 'discovered' by Essex – HTLV-4 and STLV-3. Their article, which appeared in *Nature* in 1988, made it clear that neither HTLV-4 nor STLV-3 was an 'authentic' virus. They both derived from samples of the macaque virus. All three viruses were one and the same. Essex and Kanki had to agree. The macaque virus had somehow contaminated two cultures, one containing cells from the Senegalese prostitutes and the other of cells from the African green monkey.

Carel Mulder, professor of molecular genetics at the University of Massachusetts, wrote in *Nature*: 'This episode should serve as a strong warning for all virologists working with multiple isolates [viruses] to check any new isolates against viruses present in the laboratory. I am aware, or have been told, of at least five instances in other laboratories in the United States and Europe where non-infected cell cultures became infected with HIV-1 in the same containment hood.' (A containment hood is a standard piece of laboratory equipment: an extractor removes air from the containment hood so that this air does not pass into the laboratory.)

Although Essex's African green monkey virus turned out not to be genuine, other researchers, from Japan, did find a virus that infects wild African green monkeys. This virus is called SIV_{agm}. (The SIV stands for simian immunodeficiency virus.) This virus does not seem to cause disease in wild African green monkeys. By contrast, the virus which the New England primate centre discovered in macaques – named SIV_{mac} – has been found only in captive animals, in which it causes an AIDS-like syndrome. There is no evidence that

229

wild macaques, which live in Asia, are infected with a similar virus. So the infected macaques probably caught this virus in captivity from an unknown source.

During the late 1980s, other groups of researchers isolated further simian retroviruses. In addition to SIV_{agm} and SIV_{mac}, there is also an SIV_{sm} isolated from healthy sooty mangabey monkeys. This virus causes an AIDS-like syndrome when inoculated into an unrelated monkey, the rhesus macaque. Retroviruses have also been isolated from mandrills, baboons, stump-tailed macaques, pig-tailed macaques and the cyno-molgus monkey. Perhaps most interesting of all, however, is the report of a virus which closely resembles HIV-1, which has been isolated from a chimpanzee in Gabon.

Given that the genetic sequences of many of these viruses are not available at the time of writing, it is difficult to say how these viruses are related to each other and what they tell us about their ancestry. The Japanese researchers who isolated and studied the African green monkey virus said that this virus belonged to the same group as HIV-1, HIV-2 and SIV_{mac}. However, SIV_{agm} was no more closely related to HIV-2 and SIV_{mac} than it was to HIV-1.

The fact that the African green monkey virus does not cause disease in its host would suggest that this virus had infected this species for some considerable time: the host had adapted to the virus. Some scientists have suggested that the simian immunodeficiency viruses are, indeed, very old. Mulder, in 1988, said: 'The fact that the [African green monkey virus] is so remarkably different from the human AIDS viruses indicates that the human viruses cannot have originated from African green monkeys in recent times, as had been predicted by many people. This claim was usually based on what was very probably a case of mistaken identity [Essex's mix-up].' As an intriguing afterthought, Mulder even suggests that these viruses – the African green monkey one and the HIVs – may have been present 'in the common ancestor of Old World primates and humans and have evolved along with them'.

When scientists have managed to isolate as many retro-viruses as possible from monkeys in the wild, and determined their genetic sequences, they will be able to say with rather more certainty how these viruses are related, both to each other and to the human immunodeficiency viruses. There is no doubt in the minds of most scientists that a whole range of simian retroviruses is waiting to be discovered. It is also conceivable that more related viruses – some of which may not cause AIDS – will yet be uncovered in humans.

One theory about the origin of the human immunodeficiency viruses does indeed hold that the HIVs may have existed as harmless passenger viruses which did not cause disease. In support of this idea is the discovery by researchers from the Pasteur Institute in Paris and the Center for International Medical Research in Gabon of an unusual variety of HIV which does not appear to cause AIDS. According to a report in *Science* in 1988, this virus seems to be quite widespread in Cameroon, the Congo, Gabon and the Central African Republic. This virus seemed to be very similar to HIV-1 in its genetic structure, except that it had lost its ability to produce the protein made from the *tat* gene (see p. 160). Without the *tat* product, the virus was unable to stimulate the production of its other proteins. Only a very minor change in the genetic sequence of the virus accounted for this inability. This also means, of course, that only a very minor mutation would be necessary for the virus to become able to cause disease.

Research has shown that about three people in every 200 screened for this virus in Gabon have antibodies to it, but none of them has developed AIDS. By contrast, only one person in every 200 screened for HIV-1 seems to be infected with HIV-1. By 1988, there had been at least twenty cases of AIDS in Gabon in people with antibodies to HIV-1. If people infected with the variant virus continue to remain well, this could support the idea that a related virus may have been present in human populations for a long time without causing disease.

Another theory about the origin of AIDS holds that the virus may have been present in some isolated population for many years, but began to spread only when people began to move to the cities. In 1988, some researchers presented evidence in the *New England Journal of Medicine* that this could have been the case. They studied people living in the remote Equateur province of north-west Zaïre, who had given blood samples in 1976 for a study of another viral disease, Ebola haemorrhagic fever, which broke out at that time. The samples had been stored. In 1985, the researchers tested them for antibodies to HIV. Five of the samples – fewer than one in a hundred – was positive, and HIV was isolated from one of these.

The researchers went back to the same area in 1986 and tried to trace the five individuals who had been infected. Three of them had died of illnesses suggestive of AIDS; two were healthy but still had antibodies to HIV. Four of the five individuals had never travelled outside their home area.

The researchers also tested almost 400 residents in the area and found again that fewer than one in a hundred was infected with HIV. (In almost 300 prostitutes, however, more than 10 per cent were infected.) The fact that the prevalence of infection with HIV had remained similar throughout a period of ten years suggested to the scientists that 'HIV infection and AIDS could have existed and remained stable in a rural area of Africa for a long period'. They concluded: 'Our findings suggest that the traditional village life in the Equateur province carries a low risk of HIV infection. The disruption of traditional life styles and the social and behavioural changes that accompany urbanization may be important factors in the spread of AIDS in Central Africa.'

So perhaps HIV did exist undetected for a long while in a remote area of Africa. A British researcher, Robin Weiss, of the Chester Beatty Laboratories in London, talking of the origin of HIV and AIDS at a lecture to the Royal Society in London in November 1987, quoted Pliny: '*Ex Africa semper aliquod novi*' – Out of Africa, always something new. Weiss said: 'This has offended some of our African colleagues, who dislike having the origin of AIDS placed at their feet, but I think it is probably true, and it is not intended as any sort of reproach to those countries suffering the worst impact of AIDS.'

There is, however, little clear-cut evidence that HIV was present in Africa long before it appeared elsewhere. AIDS appeared almost simultaneously in the US, Haiti, Africa and Europe, during 1980–81. African doctors are sure that if cases of AIDS had appeared earlier in any numbers, they would have noticed them. Doctors in Uganda reported in 1985 that there had been a few cases of the atypical form of Kaposi's sarcoma as far back as 1962, 'and this could suggest that AIDS has been present since then'. Yet studies such as that by Saxinger, which suggested that in the early 1970s over 60 per cent of children in the West Nile district of Uganda had antibodies to HIV, have been proved wrong. Tests in 1986 on elderly people in Kampala, and on healthy adults from the West Nile district of Uganda, showed that none and fewer than 2 per cent respectively had antibodies to HIV. These results suggested that the disease had arrived in Uganda only recently.

Other researchers have tested blood samples from over 6,000 people from nine African countries, including Zaïre, Uganda and Kenya, which had been taken and stored between 1976 and 1984. Only four samples contained antibodies to HIV. These scientists said: 'Our data do not support (nor do they totally disprove) an African origin for the human immunodeficiency virus. They do show that the virus has not been endemic in rural areas of sub-Saharan Africa until recently.' Another group of scientists tested over 1,200 blood samples which had been taken from people in Central Africa years before, about 800 of them taken as long ago as 1959. The researchers found antibodies suggestive of HIV infection in just one sample taken from someone in Leopoldville (now Kinshasa) in 1959. Even if the virus was present at that time, it certainly was not all that common.

A search for early cases of AIDS has gone on throughout the world. Retrospective studies have identified some individuals who appeared to have died of a syndrome similar to AIDS before the epidemic began. In Haiti, cases date back to

1978. In Zaïre, there seemed to have been probable cases of AIDS in 1976 and 1977.

Cases of AIDS had also occurred in Europe before the epidemic became widely apparent. One was a Spanish homosexual man who fell ill in mid-1981. Although he had a regular sexual partner, he had had sexual intercourse with other men in New York in 1974 and in Turkey in 1980. Another case that sounded like AIDS had occurred in a male homosexual violinist who had travelled widely in Europe, where he had many sexual contacts. As far as his doctors knew, he had not travelled to the US, Haiti or Africa. He fell ill in December 1976, and died of his disease in early 1979. And of the first twenty-nine cases of AIDS in France, doctors had seen nine before June 1981, when the first report of the syndrome appeared in the US. The earliest case was a thirty-one-year-old French homosexual man who had not travelled abroad in the five years before diagnosis. Doctors had diagnosed his Kaposi's sarcoma in 1974. Other reports of likely cases of AIDS came from Denmark in 1981.

In 1988, Norwegian doctors published a paper in the *Lancet* describing AIDS in a Norwegian family in the mid-1960s. The father was a sailor and had visited foreign countries, including African ports, several times before 1966. He had contracted sexually transmitted diseases on two occasions during that period. At the age of twenty, in 1966, he began to fall ill with symptoms typical of AIDS. He died in 1976. His wife began to suffer a range of infections from 1967 onwards. She also died, with symptoms typical of AIDS, in 1976. The couple had three children. Two of them, born before 1967, were healthy. The third child was born in 1967 and fell ill in 1969. She, too, died in 1976. Recent tests on stored samples of blood serum from the three patients have shown that all three were positive for HIV-1 antibodies. The two elder daughters, however, were not infected.

In the US, most early cases of AIDS (most of them in homosexual men) have dated back to about 1976. By analysing the dates of birth of children who had developed AIDS transmitted from their mothers, researchers have also found that HIV was present in heterosexual women using intravenous drugs in New York as early as 1977. According to one doctor in the US, one of his patients, a man from Haiti, died with symptoms typical of AIDS in 1959. By late 1988, scientists at the Centers for Disease Control were still studying the evidence from stored samples of this man's tissue, and had not confirmed whether this was, indeed, a case of AIDS.

One early death in the US from AIDS, however, has been confirmed by recent laboratory tests on stored tissue samples. This was a black teenager who fell ill in 1968 in St Louis, Missouri, at the age of fifteen. He died the next year. Known as Robert R., he developed swollen lymph glands, lost weight and suffered severe infections. He also had Kaposi's sarcoma. Doctors were so curious about his death that they froze samples of his blood and tissue. In 1988, the researchers published the results of their tests in the *Journal of the American Medical Association*. They said there was some evidence that the boy, who admitted being sexually active, may have been homosexual. Tests showed that he was infected with a strain of the virus which was closely related to strains of HIV-1 currently present in the US.

The researchers, commenting on the results, said that HIV or a closely related retrovirus may have been 'sporadic, episodic or even endemic' in the US at least ten years before the current epidemic. They added: 'This possibility is supported by reports, which have appeared intermittently from 1902 to 1966, describing young, non-African men with aggressive disseminated Kaposi's sarcoma, a marker suggestive of AIDS in this population . . . If a virus related to HIV has been present in the US, Africa or elsewhere for several decades, its failure to spread in an epidemic fashion earlier may reflect either a recent genetic change in the virus and/or socio-cultural factors involving sexual practices or numbers of sexual partners.'

We will probably never know where HIV came from. Many researchers believe that investigations into the origin of the virus would divert valuable resources and energy away from the real problem. What is important now, they say, is to combat the epidemic and not stand around wondering where it came from.

Chapter 13

A HETEROSEXUAL EPIDEMIC?

One of the most difficult questions that people in developed countries have asked scientists is: 'Will there be an epidemic of AIDS in heterosexuals?' The question is easy to answer on one level. There is already an epidemic in heterosexuals. In fact, heterosexual transmission is probably the commonest means of transmission of HIV. The heterosexual epidemic is already huge in Africa, but relatively small in the developed countries, being confined there largely to intravenous drug users. Although injecting drugs may be the way in which these people became infected with HIV, their sexual preferences reflect those of the general population: they are, in the main, heterosexual. They can pass the virus on to their sexual partners. It is from this group that HIV has the potential to spread into the wider heterosexual population in developed countries, although infected bisexual men may also play a role.

There is no doubt that HIV can spread by heterosexual intercourse. Women have become infected with the virus following artificial insemination with semen from an infected donor. This evidence lends support to the observations that some people have become infected after just one (sometimes two) instances of sexual intercourse with an infected partner. According to a case reported in 1987 in West Germany, a man became infected with HIV after having sex only twice with

237

an infected woman. One British study also identified two women who had become infected after just one sexual encounter with an infected partner. One of these women had had only one previous sexual partner; she caught the virus from an infected European intravenous drug user. The other had had intercourse with a man who had heterosexual contacts in Central Africa.

Studies of couples where one partner is infected, however, have shown that transmission is by no means inevitable. Some such couples can have unprotected sex for years without the infected partner succumbing to the virus. There are many theories to explain why this should be so. One possibility is that the virus may have entered the cells of the apparently uninfected partner, without stimulating that person's immune system to produce antibodies (see p. 114). Only the polymerase chain reaction test (see p. 79) would be able to diagnose these people as infected. Another theory is that people exposed to the virus who nevertheless remain uninfected may have mounted an immune response to fend it off.

There is increasing evidence, however, that infected individuals vary widely in their infectivity – in other words, in their ability to infect others. Some people may simply be good transmitters, analogous to the 'Typhoid Marys' of the nineteenth century. Clusters of HIV infection have been reported where one highly sexually active person has infected many others over a period of years. There have also been cases of individuals who have infected one sexual partner but not a later one, suggesting that infectivity changes with time.

Some researchers have suggested that a person's infectivity may alter with the course of the disease. One theory is that there are two periods of infectiousness, one shortly after infection and another beginning with the onset of AIDS. At the moment, however, scientists have no way of measuring someone's infectivity, although some researchers believe that this may correlate with the appearance of vital antigen in the blood (see p. 127). Such variation is not unknown in other diseases. In another viral disease, hepatitis B, for example, people with a certain antigen from this virus in their blood are highly infectious, compared to those who have only antibody.

Studies of couples where one partner is infected have also looked at factors such as duration of the relationship, frequency of sexual intercourse, and different sexual practices. Because HIV infection in heterosexuals is still relatively rare in developed countries, many of these studies have involved only small numbers of couples, which makes their results (some of which are conflicting) difficult to interpret. Some studies, for example, have found that the risk of transmission increases with the frequency of sexual contact and the length of the relationship. Others have found no such link. For example, researchers from the Centers for Disease Control studied more than a hundred heterosexual couples where one partner was infected. They found that one woman became infected after just one act of sexual intercourse, and another woman became infected after eight occasions. Yet eleven wives and five husbands remained uninfected after more than 200 acts of sexual intercourse with their infected spouses.

Other factors that may influence transmission of the virus include different sexual practices. One American study found that an uninfected woman was more likely to catch the virus from her infected male sexual partner if they practised anal intercourse (compared to those who had had only vaginal intercourse). However, these researchers emphasized that anal intercourse was not required in order for transmission to occur. Again, other studies have found no link between heterosexual anal intercourse and transmission to an uninfected partner. It has been difficult to determine a link between oral sex and transmission of the virus because most heterosexual couples who practise oral sex also have vaginal intercourse.

Studies designed to determine the risk of transmission from men to women and vice versa have produced conflicting results. Some studies have found that about 10 per cent of the female sexual partners of infected male haemophiliacs have become infected, too, although studies of infected people from other risk groups have sometimes shown much higher rates of transmission.

One study of people infected by contaminated blood transfusions found that 22 per cent of the wives of infected men had become infected, compared to just 8 per cent of the husbands of infected women. This fits with the idea that men 'inoculate' their sexual partners with several millilitres of infected semen, whereas men are likely to retain little infected vaginal fluid following intercourse. These biological considerations probably explain why, in gonorrhoea, the probability of a woman catching the disease from an infected man as a result of one act of intercourse is estimated to be 50:50. In the reverse direction, the risk is probabably about 25 per cent.

Other studies, however, have suggested that the likelihood of heterosexual transmission is similar in both directions. One piece of research in 1987 found that, over a three-year period, 42 per cent of the husbands and 38 per cent of the wives became HIV-positive as a result of sexual contact with their infected partners. This study contradicts the idea that it is easier for the virus to pass from men to women. Research into transmission from women to men has suffered, however, from a shortage of couples to study: few women in developed countries are infected.

Other factors which probably influence the risk of the virus passing from one person to another during sex include, for example, the presence of breaks in the skin of the genitals, particularly genital ulcers, and the presence of other sexually transmitted diseases. Lack of circumcision may also assist the virus in infecting a man. Proof that such factors play a role in the transmission of HIV comes mainly from Africa. However, one study has shown that homosexual men in the US who had had syphilis (which can cause genital ulcers) were more likely to be infected with HIV. It seems likely that the same factors play a similar role in assisting heterosexual transmission in the developed countries.

Some researchers have put together much of the available evidence on transmission of HIV in order to estimate the probability of catching HIV from an infected partner, or from a single act of intercourse with an infected person. Norman Hearst and Stephen Hulley, from the University of California, San Francisco, published their calculations in 1988 in the *Journal of the American Medical Association*. They estimated the risks associated with all kinds of situations, such as having sex with an infected partner without using condoms, and having sex with a person with no history of high-risk behaviour, with and without condoms.

Not surprisingly, the least risky activity was heterosexual intercourse with a partner with no known high-risk behaviour – and using a condom. The chance of picking up the virus under such circumstances was one in five billion for a single sexual encounter. They put the risk higher as the number of sexual encounters increased. The risk of catching HIV became one in five million for people who failed to wear condoms during sex. 'For example, the risk of AIDS from a low-risk sexual encounter is about the same as the risk of being killed in a traffic accident while driving ten miles on the way to that encounter,' Hearst and Hulley said.

The chance of infection from one heterosexual encounter with an infected person was one in 500. The most risky behaviour, they estimated, was having repeated heterosexual sex with HIV-positive partners. Even with a condom, the risk is one in eleven, they said. Without a condom, the risk rose to two in three. Condoms are not foolproof devices, they pointed out – the failure rate of condoms in preventing pregnancies can be about 10 per cent a year.

Hearst and Hulley suggested that for most sexually transmitted diseases – but not AIDS – the cumulative probability of becoming infected approaches the probability, that the partner is infected after the first few contacts. 'For an agent with very low infectivity, like HIV, on the other hand, the cumulative probability of becoming infected does not approach the probability that the partner is infected until the number of exposures to the same individual is in the hundreds. Stated differently, having sex 100 times (the number of times most young couples have sex in a year) with a partner who has a 1 per cent chance of being infected with HIV carries nearly the same risk as having sex one time each with 100 different partners who average a 1 per cent chance of being infected.'

This analysis, the first serious attempt to assess the risk of heterosexual encounters, is by no means perfect. The researchers used group averages, and chose to ignore the wider variations within groups. This can affect risk for particular individuals in certain areas, in certain circumstances. For example, as many as one in a hundred pregnant, black, non-drug-using women in Brooklyn may be infected with HIV. Other groups in other cities will have different prevalences of infection.

Hearst and Hulley's study also suffered from lack of data. In 1988, there was still not enough information on heterosexual infection with HIV to make cast-iron conclusions on risk. Another problem was the assumptions the researchers made, such as the infectivity of HIV itself. These assumptions could easily be wrong. Yet another difficulty is that although the estimate of risks may be fairly accurate at the time the data were compiled, what about the future, when HIV has spread further in certain groups within the population, for example heterosexual drug users? The risks would then increase for the heterosexual population as a whole.

Several groups of researchers wrote to the journal criticizing this paper. One letter pointed out that Hearst and Hulley had concluded that 'the single most important message for patients is to have sex only with partners who they know are at low risk of carrying HIV infection'. Yet, the authors of the letter said, people working in the field of AIDS have consistently found that even experienced interviewers find it difficult to extract sensitive information on high-risk behaviour from people presenting with HIV infection. 'To expect such skills to become part of selecting a sexual partner is impractical.' These researchers also pointed out that 'the consequences of HIV infection are so profound that even a remote risk of infection should be minimized'.

Other correspondents identified similar drawbacks. What

242

about people who had practised high-risk behaviour in the past but since stopped, they asked. One researcher reported the case of a woman whose fourth child, the first of her second marriage, was found to be infected with HIV. Investigations showed that her second husband was a former intravenous drugs user who had stopped using drugs before the couple met. 'Even with the intimacy of marriage and childbirth,' the letter said, 'the wife had never ascertained that her husband was at high risk of HIV infection.'

Some scientists, such as Roy Anderson from Imperial College in London, suggest that the most important factor in assessing the risk of a heterosexual epidemic is the rate of partner change within the heterosexual population. From surveys of sexual behaviour, Anderson has estimated that some heterosexuals have one or two partners, on average, per year, whereas some homosexuals – at least in the early 1980s, when AIDS was barely heard of – may have an average of ten different partners a year. Anderson has suggested that the rate of partner change which could trigger an epidemic in heterosexuals might be about five a year. Some heterosexuals do have as many partners in a year as this, and therefore a heterosexual epidemic could well occur, albeit at a much slower pace than the epidemic in homosexuals that began in the early 1980s. Such an epidemic, Anderson suggested in a paper published in *Nature* in 1988, could have a doubling time in its early stages of eight to fourteen years – far slower than the doubling time of about one year in the early stages of the AIDS epidemic in homosexuals. Anderson has pointed out: 'The disease may be spreading 10 times more slowly among heterosexuals than among homosexuals because they have 10 times fewer partners. If that is so then the AIDS epidemic may be expected to take 10 times as long to peak in the heterosexual population.' There will be a very slow rise in the number of HIV positives in the general population, Anderson said, 'on a timescale of decades'.

What is the evidence that AIDS is spreading into the wider heterosexual population? Information on this aspect is very patchy. Some studies, according to their authors, seem to

243

suggest that HIV is hardly spreading at all among heterosexuals. In 1988, for example, one London doctor who specializes in genitourinary medicine put the case against a heterosexual epidemic. 'There is scarcely any evidence that sex between heterosexuals poses a risk of AIDS, even when a number of partners are involved. It is deception to suggest otherwise.' The doctor, Brian Evans of the West London Hospital, was speaking after completing a survey of 3,000 women who had attended the hospital's clinic for sexually transmitted diseases. The women were heterosexual and, of course, sexually active – probably more so than the general population, given that they had sought medical treatment.

The clinic was also in an area with a large number of homosexual and bisexual men infected with HIV, so the women were at a higher-than-usual risk of coming into contact with infected bisexual men. Evans argued that these women were the very group of heterosexuals most at risk of AIDS. He found that seven of the women were infected with the virus; all of them had partners who were either bisexual or injected drugs. 'It is very encouraging,' he said at the time, 'that despite all the fears, HIV infection does not appear to be spreading into heterosexuals.'

Another study, this time looking at almost 2,000 prostitutes in New York, also seemed to support the contention that AIDS was not spreading via heterosexual contact. Researchers found that about 12 per cent of the women in these studies were infected with HIV but nearly all of them had a history of intravenous drug use. (These figures were in stark contrast to the proportion of prostitutes who are infected in some cities of East Africa, which rose from fewer than 10 per cent in 1981 to more than 80 per cent in 1988.) Investigations found that the prostitutes in New York had become infected by sharing contaminated needles and syringes rather than through heterosexual contact with infected clients. Researchers who interviewed more than 600 male clients of the prostitutes found fewer than a handful who had become infected with HIV.

Studies such as these seemed to back the belief that heterosexual AIDS on a massive scale is an unlikely prospect for the West. Other studies, however, did not support this thesis. At almost the same time that Evans was reassuring the British heterosexual population, another London doctor, Michael Adler, a professor of genitourinary medicine at the Middlesex Hospital, was putting forward the opposing viewpoint. 'At the start, there seemed to be special factors about the African epidemic which lulled people into thinking that a similar pattern would not happen in the UK,' he said. 'But the comforting thought that African AIDS is special to Africa has now been discredited.'

So even in 1988, seven years after doctors diagnosed the first cases of AIDS, the experts were still divided on the question of a heterosexual epidemic in the developed countries. Many people began to suspect that some scientists were exaggerating the risk to heterosexuals in order to ensure that the largely heterosexual public would keep the pressure on governments to spend more money on AIDS research. There was convincing evidence, however, that a heterosexual epidemic was under way in developed countries. This evidence came largely from studies in the US, the first country to realize that it had a problem with AIDS in homosexuals.

When scientists began to study the figures of AIDS cases in the US for 1985 and 1986, they found that the category of heterosexuals – without any other risk behaviour, such as injecting intravenous drugs – was growing faster than any other group. At the end of 1985, the number of heterosexuals with AIDS had grown by 130 per cent. By the end of 1986, the figure had swollen by 145 per cent, compared to a growth rate of about 60 or 70 per cent for AIDS cases in general. The absolute figure for heterosexuals with AIDS was still small, about 4 per cent of the total. Nevertheless, the rate of growth was very high. Heterosexually transmitted AIDS, which accounted for just 1 per cent of all cases in late 1983, accounted for 3.5 per cent of cases in 1988. The same year, one leading researcher said it looked as though the figure would rise to 10 per cent in less than a decade.

One way of studying the problem is to look at the time it

takes for the number of AIDS cases in a particular group to double. In 1988, scientists estimated that this so-called 'doubling time' for heterosexual cases of AIDS in the US was about eleven months. This was shorter than the current doubling time for AIDS in homosexuals, but approximately the same as the doubling time had been in the early 1980s, when, in the US, AIDS was almost exclusively a disease of homosexuals. Jeffrey Harris, pofessor of economics at the Massachusetts Institute of Technology, estimated that if the 1988 doubling time continued unchanged, it would result in 85,000 cases of AIDS in heterosexuals in the US by 1993. 'Accordingly,' he said in 1988, 'the first key indicator to watch is the doubling time of heterosexual AIDS cases. If there is really no impending epidemic of heterosexual AIDS, then this doubling time should soon start to rise.'

In Europe, the penetration of AIDS into heterosexuals in 1988 was not as advanced as in the US, save for certain areas. In Belgium, for instance, a high proportion of AIDS cases were in heterosexuals – more than 20 per cent. Virtually all of them had had heterosexual contact with Africans in or from the former Belgian colonies. Peter Piot, from the Institute of Tropical Medicine in Antwerp, said in 1987 that Belgium 'seems to be at the crossroads between Africa and Europe for patterns of AIDS transmission . . . Virtually all heterosexual patients were probably infected in Africa or by people who had been sexually active in Africa.'

As in the US, those parts of Europe that had a high number of intravenous drug users who shared needles and syringes also had relatively high numbers of heterosexuals with AIDS. The problem was particularly acute in Italy, which has a high number of heroin addicts. In Scotland, more than half of the HIV-positive people diagnosed up to September 1988 were known to inject drugs. Almost 30 per cent of these individuals – more than four times the national average for Britain – were women, and eighty-one people had become infected by heterosexual contact with infected drug users by mid-1988. Although these figures were small compared to those for the cities such as New York, the proportion of heterosexual cases was well above the national average for Britain. 'I don't think we can prevent spread into the heterosexual population,' said Ray Brettle, from Edinburgh City Hospital, 'because it's already there.'

The next obvious question, of course, is how will we know the extent to which HIV is penetrating the wider population, given that this virus takes, on average, about eight years to cause AIDS? The only way to find out would be to begin widespread screening. Screening for HIV must not be confused with mandatory testing with the aim of discriminating against people who are positive, as proposed by President Reagan in his first public speech on AIDS and practised by many countries, such as the US, the USSR, South Africa and Cuba. Screening can be completely anonymous: the blood sample need carry no identifying marks that would allow the result to be connected to the person who gave the blood. Such screening provides only information on the extent to which the virus is spreading in selected populations. There is no need, therefore, to know the names of the people involved, although it is useful to know something about their background, such as their sexual preferences.

In Britain, the government resisted arguments that began in 1986 for widescale screening of the heterosexual population. The problem was partly the question of ethics. The government was worried that it would be seen to be condoning the mandatory testing of people's blood. Nevertheless, at the end of 1988 the first pilot schemes began for testing the blood of pregnant women attending antenatal clinics. The government decided that these women were a good group to test because they are sexually active, they are heterosexual and they already give blood for a variety of other reasons. The government stopped short of a completely anonymous and compulsory screening programme, however. Instead, doctors asked the women whether they would volunteer to have the test, and offered them the opportunity of knowing the result. Many scientists dislike this way of conducting a screening programme on the grounds that even if only a tiny minority opt out, these could be the very people most likely to be infected

– a serious source of bias. In the event, scientific opinion in favour of fully anonymous screening forced the government to make a U-turn. In October 1988, the Secretary of State for Health, Kenneth Clarke, ordered the introduction of a scheme to screen people attending hospitals and clinics.

In the US at the end of 1987, health authorities in New York City began a screening programme which would eventually involve about 20,000 newborn infants. The programme revealed that one in every sixty-one babies born in the city carried antibodies to HIV. This does not necessarily mean that the babies themselves are infected because the antibodies could have come from the mother and passed to the fetus in the womb. But at least one in sixty-one mothers in the survey must be infected with HIV, because only 25 to 50 per cent of babies born to infected mothers show signs of infection. In parts of the city, for example the Bronx, the incidence was much higher – one in forty-three newborn babies. The US has since extended the screening of newborn infants. Scientists say that a third of the babies born in the US during 1989 will be tested anonymously for HIV antibody, which will mean testing almost four million babies in all. Other screening programmes have also begun in the US on pregnant women attending antenatal clinics, people attending clinics for sexually transmitted diseases, and military recruits.

Screening studies such as these indicate that AIDS is already a serious problem in poor, inner city areas of the US where injection of intravenous drugs is widespread. The problem is also becoming a problem of poverty and racial background. All screening studies of heterosexuals in the US find that blacks and Hispanics are far more likely to be HIV-positive than whites. The results of a screening programme in the American armed forces, which began in January 1986, found that, among active-service personnel, blacks were 3.6 times and Hispanics 2.5 times more likely to be infected with the virus than whites. Although blacks and Hispanics constitute about 51 per cent of those who were found to be HIV positive, they represent only 23 per cent of all active-service personnel. This screening programme, which is part of the mandatory testing regime introduced by President Reagan, shows that the prevalence of the virus among American service personnel is 1.3 per 1,000. This is remarkably high, given that people with high-risk behaviour are discouraged from joining the armed forces, and are tested for HIV infection before they can join.

By mid-1988, blacks and Hispanics accounted for 70 per cent of the cases of AIDS in heterosexual men, 70 per cent in women and 75 per cent in children. A large majority of these adults were regular users of intravenous drugs. It became clear to those fighting AIDS that the battle against a heterosexual epidemic is also a battle against the use of intravenous drugs. Researchers are convinced that if a heterosexual epidemic takes off, it will begin with the closed communities of intravenous drug users where education and prevention can be acutely difficult.

Wider screening programmes and more research into the factors influencing transmission of the virus will clear up many of the questions surrounding the prospects of an epidemic in heterosexuals. One issue to bear in mind is how wide does the spread have to be before it is called an epidemic? Even if only 1 per cent of heterosexuals in developed countries become infected and eventually develop AIDS, the implications for health services are enormous.

Practically the only consensus to emerge by 1988, however, was that it is still too early to determine whether there will be a massive epidemic of AIDS in heterosexuals in the developed world to mirror what has happened in heterosexuals in Africa and in gay men. Jeffrey Harris of the Massachusetts Institute of Technology asked the question in 1988, and felt confident to predict: 'If it is going to happen at all, my hunch is that we'll know within the next two years. In the meantime, the potential for a megaton epidemic remains.'

Chapter 14

WASTED YEARS

Economists say that when America sneezes, Europe catches a cold. Those who study AIDS may notice a parallel. This time, however, America sneezed and nobody took any notice. While the US became riddled with pneumonia – quite literally – Europe began to feel a chill.

The story of AIDS, as far as the US is concerned, is one of missed opportunity. America has more documented cases of AIDS, by far, than any other country in the developed world. The US realized before anywhere else that it had an AIDS epidemic on its hands. It had had ample warnings of an impending catastrophe, and the technical means and money to take the necessary evasive action and educate its public. Yet the US government, unlike many European governments, has shown an astonishing lack of direction in tackling what senior health advisers have labelled the biggest public-health problem of the twentieth century.

While European governments have fought AIDS with the only effective weapon there is at present – education campaigns – the US government prevaricated and procrastinated beyond belief. And yet, the scale of the tragedy in the US is massive. By the end of 1988, nearly 100,000 Americans had developed AIDS. More than a quarter of a million Americans will have suffered from AIDS by 1991. Even this might be an underestimate of the true tally. In 1986, the Centers for

Disease Control predicted 15,800 new cases in that year, and 23,000 new cases for 1987. In fact, there were 17,100 new cases in 1986 and 25,200 in 1987.

In September 1988, the US government estimated that there would be 365,000 cases of AIDS diagnosed in the US by the end of 1992, with 263,000 deaths. In 1992 alone, the government expects doctors to diagnose 80,000 new cases and to write death certificates for 66,000 more. The bill for the health care of AIDS patients in that year alone could be anything between $5 billion and $13 billion. The problem for the US is going to be tremendous, and stands as a warning for the rest of the developed world.

Governments in Europe have had the advantage of being able to learn something from the American experience of AIDS. But the US government itself has been slow to catch on. Governments in Europe were preparing for their second or third wave of health education campaigns at the same time that the US government had barely embarked on its own nationally coordinated effort. In 1987, for instance, the US was still deliberating over plans to send education leaflets to American households. When it did, in the middle of 1988, many Americans had no doubt become infected with HIV in that year as a result of ignorance or complacency.

The Reagan administration, which sat through seven years of the American epidemic, must share much of the responsibility for delaying the prevention of this human disaster. Ronald Reagan himself has much to answer for. His first public speech specifically about AIDS – before a glittering dinner at the Potomac Hotel in Washington DC in May 1987 – was littered with misguided intentions. The emphasis he chose for his fight against AIDS is extraordinary for its blind faith in technology's ability to solve the problem and its preoccupation with mandatory testing.

On that evening of 31 May 1987, six years after scientists had first found AIDS in groups of homosexual men in California, Reagan had finally summoned up the political courage to talk about the disease. He told his audience of scientists, dignatories and film stars:

Just as most individuals don't know they carry the virus, no one knows to what extent the virus has infected our entire society. AIDS is surreptitiously spreading throughout our population, and yet we have no accurate measure of its scope. It is time we knew exactly what we were facing. And this is why I support routine testing.

I have asked the Department of Health and Human Services [HSS] to determine as soon as possible the extent to which the AIDS virus has penetrated our society and to predict its future dimensions.

I have also asked the HHS to add the AIDS virus to the list of contagious diseases for which immigrants and aliens seeking permanent residence in the United States can be denied entry.

I have asked the Department of Justice to plan for testing all Federal prisoners, as well as looking into ways to protect uninfected inmates and their families.

In addition, I've asked for a review of other Federal responsibilities, such as veterans' hospitals, to see if testing might be appropriate in these areas. This is in addition to the testing already under way in our military and foreign service.

For good measure, Reagan added that he would encourage states to 'offer' routine testing for those people seeking marriage licences. 'I would like to think,' he said, 'that everyone getting married would want to be tested.' Reagan's audience, save for a few scientists, applauded his pronouncement. His vice-president, George Bush, did not receive such a polite response a day later, when he delivered the same message at the opening of the Third International Conference on AIDS. His statements that 'there must be more testing' met with derision from many in the audience of scientists. Now Bush, as President, must take responsibility for the future fight against AIDS.

There are grave problems with mandatory testing for infection with HIV in order to discriminate against individuals. To start with, there are technical problems: the test cannot be 100 per cent accurate. Another difficulty is the long period of latency between infection with the virus and the appearance of the antibodies identified by the test. In addition, and most important of all, people need to ask what will be gained by mandatory and routine testing of large groups of the popu-

252

lation who are not at any special risk of AIDS. To a great extent, the tests become more accurate with high-risk groups, where the virus is more prevalent. Testing the population at large, therefore, for no obvious reason other than 'the government says it must be done' merely compounds the problems raised by the test.

Even before Reagan made his speech, the World Health Organization had already addressed some of these difficulties. A month previously, the WHO had published a report on routine screening of foreign visitors. The WHO identified a major problem with testing large numbers of international travellers. Suppose, the WHO said, that in a group of 1 million travellers, there are 10,000 (1 per cent) who are carriers for the virus, in other words true HIV positives. The rest, 990,000 are true negatives. Now suppose that an immigration authority of a country began testing these 1 million visitors with a blood test that could identify true positives 99 per cent of the time (its 'sensitivity', as described in Chapter 5). The test would find 9,900 of the true positives, but fail to identify 100 carriers of the virus, who would be free to visit the country in question. If the same test could accurately identify true negatives 99 per cent of the time (its 'specificity'), then the test would correctly label 980,100 out of 990,000 true negatives. Furthermore, it would wrongly classify 9,900 negative people as HIV positive.

So, in this hypothetical situation the test would label 19,800 people as positive. But half are true positives, and half are false positives. In other words, the test, used to conduct mass screening without confirmatory testing, is no better than flipping a coin at predicting who is really infected with the virus that causes AIDS. Furthermore, the test has failed to identify 100 truly HIV positive people. And this is with a test that is 99 per cent specific and sensitive – most testing would be less accurate under the difficult conditions of quick mass screening of foreigners.

The WHO said that mass testing of foreign travellers 'can lead to massive misallocation of resources'. These resources:

would be more effectively directed to educating the population concerning HIV or to screening of blood for transfusion. A less obvious negative effect could be a false sense of security about seronegative travellers, leading to laxity regarding behaviours which spread the virus and an actual increase in overall risk for HIV transmission from international travellers to national residents. Finally, it is quite possible that HIV screening of international travellers, if practised on a selective geographical basis, would provide a disincentive for the reporting of AIDS, resulting in further distortion of the critical surveillance function necessary for ongoing monitoring of the world-wide epidemic.

Routine testing of foreign visitors, in other words, can be positively harmful. By the time Reagan had made his speech, the WHO had made it abundantly clear that it opposed the sort of mandatory screening programmes that he now publicly supported: 'There are more effective, less intrusive and less costly measures for preventing HIV transmission than the use of mandatory universal screening,' the WHO said.

President Reagan, however, ignored these powerful arguments against enforced screening. The US government introduced legislation in the summer of 1987 to test potential immigrants for HIV infection, although it stopped short of plans to screen tourists and those entering the US on business. The Presidential Commission on the HIV Epidemic made it clear in its report in 1988 that it did not agree with this policy. 'At best, border screening programmes would only briefly retard the spread of HIV,' it said. The commission called for the policy to be re-evaluated.

The government has, however, set aside hundreds of millions of dollars for further testing programmes elsewhere in government that had nothing directly to do with the health of the people involved. Reagan's accountants estimated that he spent $168m in 1988 on blood tests that took place outside America's health system – in the Department of Defense and Department of Labor, for instance. It is a powerful sign to private organizations that they, too, should accept the necessity of mass screening on a routine basis. Individual states,

254

notably Illinois and Louisiana, have gone ahead with their own testing programmes, primarily aimed at couples who want to get married. But the result was that many people crossed into neighbouring states that did not require an HIV test before issuing a marriage certificate. Nevertheless, for a few couples, testing for HIV proved horrendous. One woman from Chicago, for instance, was told several weeks before her marriage that she had proved to be HIV positive. Even though her doctor advised her that the result was likely to be a false positive, because she had no obvious risk behaviour, she became emotionally distraught. Such false positives can take months to disprove, by which time the psychological turmoil has the potential to destroy the prospective marriage.

America, of course, is not alone in its fascination with the test for infection with HIV. Many countries, of all political persuasions, have instigated mandatory screening programmes of one sort or another. A related issue is whether doctors have the right to test their patients for HIV infection without their patients' consent. In Britain, doctors voted at the British Medical Association's annual conference in July 1987 for secretive tests to protect themselves from possible infection. After the vote, the chairman of the BMA's council, John Marks, took legal advice. The BMA's lawyers said that testing for HIV infection without the knowledge or consent of the doctors' patients would constitute 'an invasion of the patient's bodily integrity' and is therefore grounds for the patient to sue the doctor for assault. The council quickly ruled that it would not be in the interests of the BMA to condone such surreptitious tests, and so overruled the vote of its own membership. The following year, British doctors again made it clear that they wanted to be able to test any patient for HIV without first informing that person. Hospital doctors, especially, were worried about the risks they might face in treating people who may be infected with HIV.

The American Medical Association, the equivalent of the BMA in the US, has rejected secret tests. The AMA also passed a resolution at its annual meeting in 1987 to protect the confidentiality of patients tested for HIV infection. But only, the association said, if that privacy does not infringe another person's right to safety. If a man refuses to tell his wife that he is HIV positive, then the doctor can tell her in order to protect her health. The American Medical Association takes the view that people who are HIV positive have the right to be 'free from irrational acts of prejudice', but, equally, others have the right to protection against 'an unreasonable risk of disease'.

Testing for HIV infection is therefore a balancing act between the rights of the individual and the rights of society and others at large. Two doctors from the New England Medical Center in Boston, Klemens Meyer and Stephen Pauker, summed up the dilemma and highlighted their worries over testing in an article they wrote for the *New England Journal of Medicine* in July 1987: 'We are a testing culture: we test our urine for drugs; we test our sweat for lies. It is not surprising that we should test our blood for the acquired immune deficiency syndrome.' They warned that inaccurate tests – and tests are always inaccurate to some extent – can turn a screening programme into a social catastrophe. 'An AIDS epidemic frightens us all,' they said,

but we should not allow our fear to cloud our judgement. Hasty and indiscriminate screening for antibody to HIV is imprudent and potentially dangerous, whether we suggest the tests to young women, require them of engaged couples, or impose them on our veterans . . . If we want to test each other, we should make a deliberate choice of the threshold probability of infection above which we will screen. We should make explicit the trade-offs in any testing programme. How many engagements should end to prevent one infection? How many jobs should be lost? How many insurance policies should be cancelled or denied? How many fetuses should be aborted and how many couples should remain childless to avert the birth of one child with AIDS?

Without HIV testing, it is true, the US will not know the extent to which the virus has penetrated American society. But testing need not, and should not, go hand in glove with discrimination. Truly anonymous or strictly confidential testing is the only way of ensuring that people infected with HIV do not suffer discrimination as the result of a test. With those suffering the obvious symptoms of AIDS, discrimination is more difficult to prevent. The Presidential Commission on AIDS recommended measures to curb discrimination against people with AIDS, and people infected with HIV. It also recommended a law to ensure confidentiality of HIV tests. By all accounts, the members of the commission were shocked by what they described as 'obscene incidents' of discrimination against people infected with HIV. People who fear such discrimination are avoiding tests, and the fear of what other members of society might do to infected people is driving HIV underground.

A national survey of American public opinion, published in 1988, revealed that most Americans see the AIDS epidemic as inevitably leading to more discrimination against infected people. Most Americans see control of AIDS as requiring some loss of individual privacy or restrictions on civil rights. A large minority see AIDS as a deserved punishment for offensive or immoral behaviour. Nearly one in three Americans want to see HIV-infected people tattooed so that their antibody status is there for all to see. Substantial minorities of Americans want people infected with HIV to be thrown out of their jobs, evicted from their homes, or have their infected children barred from attending school.

The opinions of typical Americans in 1988 may change as more and more people become aware of AIDS through first-hand experience. By the beginning of the 1990s, AIDS will have a much higher profile in society than it does even now. How American society will cope with the volume of infection, and how it treats its infected citizens, will be the greatest test of all.

The reluctance of some governments to tackle AIDS in a forthright way has been due in part to a refusal to acknowledge that the risks posed by the virus are real. Some people cannot accept that they, their families and their friends may be at risk. Only when the people in power realize that 'it could happen to them' do countries start to grapple seriously with the problem. Yet prejudices and taboos are still everywhere paralysing the will to act. Some parents would rather ignore the fact that their children might be sexually active than tell them how to reduce their risk of catching AIDS by using a condom. Some authorities would prefer to carry on denying drug addicts clean needles in the false assumption that this will stop addicts from injecting drugs. And some prime ministers and presidents prefer to avoid using the word 'homosexual', as if, by pretending that homosexuals did not exist, they might go away.

If governments are to stop AIDS, they must reach out to the margins of society. One way to help to stop the spread of AIDS among drug addicts, for example, is to provide them with clean needles. In some major cities, such as Edinburgh and New York, over half the drug addicts are infected. Researchers believe that the figure is so high because it is the policy of the police to search addicts, confiscating needles and syringes. The result is that many addicts are forced to share needles with others, facilitating the spread of HIV. Plans in several British cities to give addicts clean needles in return for used ones have sometimes met with resistance. Those who oppose such schemes, however, should ask which is worse: appearing to condone drug addiction by supplying the necessary equipment or turning a blind eye to a breeding ground for the virus. In 1988, the British government provided health authorities with an extra £3m to set up needle-exchange schemes, which, the government acknowledged, could help to change the behaviour of intravenous drug users. The change of policy provided a much-needed fillip to those working with this high-risk group.

Another breeding ground for the virus is sexually active heterosexuals. The 'moral majority' preach monogamy within marriage and chastity outside it. In the past, society could afford to be hypocritical about sex, pretending that youngsters stayed virgins until marriage, while knowing that this was rarely the case. It is no longer tenable for society to ignore premarital relationships. The threat of the virus gaining hold

258

in young people who are experimenting with sex is too great. Health education is the only weapon in the battle against AIDS in this vulnerable group.

Britain's health education campaign has been held up as a model to other countries – despite its dependency on inculcating fear. Critics labelled it as either tasteless or too muted, depending on their standpoint. Yet its frankness and popular approach has made 'condom' a household word. In contrast, rumour has it that the word condom became known in the White House as the 'C-word', because of President Reagan's reluctance to talk about the prophylactic.

By 1988, the world's only weapon against AIDS was prevention. In the developed countries, prevention (on the whole) equals health education. Sadly, the amount of resources being poured into developing effective ways of educating people fails to reflect the importance of this aspect of controlling AIDS. Health education is the poor relation of research into drugs and vaccines, which pulls in billions of dollars of support throughout the world. Given the evidence that health education can work – witness the fact that transmission of the virus among gay men in most major cities has virtually halted – it seems ironic that governments are not prepared to invest more in it.

In developing countries, money is not the only problem. In many such countries, a significant proportion of the population is not able to read. Even if radio and television broadcasts can reach all regions (they frequently cannot), not everyone may have access to a radio or a television. Many people also speak a different language to the one in which official broadcasts are made.

Health education programmes suitable for people living in New York will not be appropriate for inhabitants of Nairobi, for example. The message has to be adapted according to the country and the culture. Little research is going on into ways of putting over the message about AIDS in developing countries.

Health education must go hand in hand with other strategies that will prevent the spread of AIDS in developing countries. Programmes to screen donated blood, for example, are now underway in many countries in Africa. The WHO's Global Programme on AIDS has helped many countries in sub-Saharan Africa to begin screening donated blood. As a result, in many countries, the only hospital departments working properly are the blood banks. American researchers have calculated that in some countries, the cost of screening donated blood, per transfusion, costs about thirty times the annual health budget for one person.

Lack of resources also helps to spread HIV. In some countries, such as Zaïre, research has suggested that medical injections probably assist the spread of the virus. In Zaïre, the health budget for the whole country, with a population of thirty million people, is less than the budget of a British district hospital screening a tenth of this number. In Zaïre, needles are reused, often on as many as thirty people, until they break.

The problem of AIDS in developing countries calls into question the entire issue of how to deliver aid. Some researchers have called for a campaign to diagnose and treat sexually transmitted diseases, given the observation that such diseases seem to facilitate the spread of AIDS. How could such a programme work in isolation from the services that the West takes for granted: laboratory services for diagnosis, drugs for treatment, social workers to carry out contact tracing. AIDS does indeed, as the WHO is fond of saying, show up our inadequacies and highlight many injustices.

One thing is clear. No country should shirk from implementing measures to control the spread of AIDS because its government hopes that science will soon provide a 'magic bullet'. We already have cures for diseases such as syphilis and gonorrhoea. So why do so many people still suffer from these damaging infections? The first few years of the AIDS epidemic have seen a huge burst of knowledge about the virus and disease, as scientists applied their available technology to a new problem. By 1988, however, the study of AIDS was up against the boundaries of knowledge. Scientists and researchers have settled down to a long, hard slog.

Drugs will probably never provide a solution to infection with HIV. They would have to be taken for life, because the vital genetic material would always remain in the body's cells. The costs of such long-term treatment could cripple health services in many developed countries. In Africa, the annual budget for health care per person per year is unlikely to stretch to paying for even a single accurate diagnostic test for HIV infection.

Nevertheless, the prospects for a drug that would delay the onset of AIDS and perhaps prevent infected people from passing on the virus to others are somewhat better than the prospects for a vaccine. Some scientists fear that it may prove impossible to develop a vaccine to protect against HIV. And until science has an answer to AIDS, the only barrier that the virus will respect is less than a millimetre thick and made of rubber. This thin latex line may be the only way that we have of limiting the sexual transmission of AIDS.

GLOSSARY

AIDS: acquired immune deficiency syndrome, the collection of illnesses resulting from infection with the human immuno-deficiency virus, HIV. Acquired because it is not inherited; immune deficiency because the immune system is seriously weakened; and syndrome because AIDS is a collection of symptoms and illnesses.

antibodies: molecules produced by B-cells in response to an antigen. By binding to the antigen, antibodies make it easier for cells such as macrophages to engulf and eliminate the foreign particle.

antigens: foreign substances or particles such as proteins, bacteria or viruses, which cause the body to produce antibodies. Viral antigens are viral components such as viral proteins.

ARV: AIDS-related virus, one of the early names for HIV, coined by scientists working in California.

B-cells: also called B-lymphocytes. They are a special type of white blood cell that can produce antibodies.

cell-mediated immunity: important in eliminating micro-organisms such as viruses which live inside cells where anti-bodies are unable to act. It is controlled mainly by the two types of T-cell.

DNA: deoxyribonucleic acid, the genetic material which is the blueprint for living organisms.

262

ELISA: enzyme-linked immunosorbent assay, the type of blood test commonly used to detect antibodies to HIV.

envelope protein: the envelope protein of the human immunodeficiency virus is called gp160, which splits to form two smaller molecules, gp41 and gp120. The envelope protein appears on the surface of the virus.

factor VIII: the protein which is necessary for the formation of blood clots in humans.

FAIDS: feline acquired immune deficiency syndrome, AIDS in cats.

false negative: when a blood test incorrectly finds no antibodies to HIV when in reality they are present.

false positive: when a blood test incorrectly finds antibodies to HIV when in reality there are none.

gene: the single unit of inheritance, common to all living things including viruses.

genetic engineering: the technology of manipulating genetic material, usually with new techniques based on splicing and inserting DNA.

glycoproteins: proteins with sugar molecules on their surfaces. The envelope proteins of the human immunodeficiency virus are glycoproteins.

haemophilia: a blood-clotting disorder usually due to a deficiency of factor VIII.

HIV: human immunodeficiency virus, the virus that results in AIDS. Different types of HIV are called HIV-1, HIV-2, etc. An international committee of virologists decided on the name in 1986.

HIV-negative: if someone is said to be HIV-negative, they have no detectable antibodies to the virus.

HIV-positive: if someone is said to be HIV-positive, they have antibodies to the virus, they are infected with the virus, and they are capable of transmitting the virus to others.

HTLV: human T-cell leukaemia/lymphoma virus, which later became known as human T-cell lymphotropic virus. Different types are called HTLV-1, HTLV-2, etc. Robert Gallo named the AIDS virus 'HTLV-3' in 1984.

immunoglobulins: antibodies.

LAV: lymphadenopathy-associated virus, the name given by Luc Montagnier to describe the AIDS virus in 1983.

lentivirus: a type of retrovirus characterized by the slowness with which it attacks its host animal. HIV is a lentivirus.

lymphocytes: white blood cells known as T-cells and B-cells.

macrophages: large mobile cells capable of engulfing and destroying microorganisms. They also have an important role in 'presenting' antigens to T-cells.

monocytes: immature, unspecialized macrophages.

mutation: a change in the genetic material which often gives rise to a change in the appearance of an organism.

mutation rate: the speed at which mutations occur.

pandemic: an extensive epidemic affecting wide geographical areas.

p24 protein: one of the inner proteins of HIV. Its presence in the blood may be important as an early indicator of the future development of AIDS.

polymerase chain reaction (PCR) test: this test makes it possible to identify minute traces of genetic material (of HIV, for example) in a sample of tissue. The technique relies on multiplying the genetic material to a point at which scientists can detect it.

retrovirus: a type of virus that has RNA as its genetic material, rather than DNA, and which has an enzyme to make a DNA-copy of its RNA.

reverse transcriptase: the enzyme unique to HIV that controls the manufacture of viral DNA from the viral genetic material RNA.

RNA: ribonucleic acid, another type of genetic material. Living things usually make RNA-copies of DNA.

SAIDS: simian AIDS, AIDS in monkeys.

sensitivity: the probability of a blood test giving a positive result when antibodies to HIV are in fact present. Highly sensitive tests give low false negative rates.

seroconversion: the name given to the point at which someone in whom it was not previously possible to detect antibodies first produces antibodies against a microorganism.

seronegative: the status of someone who has no detectable antibodies to a particular microorganism, such as HIV.

seropositive: the status of someone who has antibodies that recognize a particular microorganism, such as HIV.

serum: the fluid that remains after the cells have been removed from the blood. It is this fluid that doctors test when they are looking for antibodies to HIV.

SIV: simian immunodeficiency virus, the group of viruses that infect monkeys, some of which can cause AIDS-like symptoms in some species.

specificity: the probability of a blood test giving a negative result when antibodies to HIV are in fact not present. Highly specific tests give low false positive rates.

T-cells: a type of white blood cell or lymphocyte. There are two main kinds of T-cell, helper cells and cytotoxic cells. The helper cells are stimulated by antigen on the surface of macrophages, and can then cause B-cells to produce antibodies, macrophages to engulf microorganisms and cytotoxic cells to destroy infected cells.

virus: one of the simplest organisms. They lead parasitic existences by hijacking the machinery of living cells.

Western blot: a type of test which is complex to perform but which is highly accurate and so is often used to confirm positive results from other, simpler tests.

INDEX

amniotic fluid 131
ampligen 163–4
amyl nitrites 25–6
anatomy of HIV 94–111
anaemia 154
anal intercourse 115, 132, 133, 239
anal warts 125
Anderson, Roy 225, 243
Angola 199, 211
antibodies 99, 262
  anti-idiotype 187–8, 189
  boosting immune system by 146
  loss of 115–16
  monoclonal 188, 190
  neutralizing 100–102, 171, 173
  tests for 35, 36–7, 64, 70, 71–4,
    84–6, 113
antibody-dependent cell-mediated
  cytotoxicity [ADCC] 171
antigens 99, 262
  cellular [HLA] 97
  epitopes 188
  'marker', in vaccines 195
  tests to detect 78, 113, 127–9
Antwerp 203–4
ARC (AIDS-related complex) 118
Armour Pharmaceuticals 91–2
artificial insemination 237
ARV (AIDS-related virus) 46, 262
Australia 90, 162
autologous transfusions 66
azidothymidine/AZT 149–56

B-cells 99–100, 101, 122, 171, 262
baculovirus 177–8, 182
Barbara, John 86
Barré-Sinoussi, Françoise 30
Barzach, Michèle 56
Bayley, Anne 202, 205–6
Benn, Steven 49
bedbugs 140–41
Belgium 198–9, 201, 203–5, 246
Belle Glade, Florida 140
Benin 199, 210
Biggar, Robert 207–9

binding site, blocking of 186–9
Biocine 183
biology of HIV 94–111
Biotech Research Laboratories 65
bisexual men 237, 244
blood
  accidental contact 140–42
  levels of virus in 114, 131
  risk from donors 135
  trade in products 63, 90–91
  transmission by 134–5, 138
  see also blood supply
Blood Products Laboratory, Elstree
  92
blood supply
  Africa 134, 198
  autologous 66
  clearing of virus 63–5, 68–70
  high-risk donors 66, 87, 88, 134
  infection from 66–8, 110–11,
    133–4, 138, 198; evidence for
    research 27–8, 110, 126
  proportion contaminated 87–8
  screening 22–3, 83–4, 134, 198,
    226, 253–4, 260
  WHO Global Programme 226
  see also: Britain; United States
blood–brain barrier 121, 123,
  144–5, 148
Bolognesi, Dani 184
bone grafts 135
bone marrow 103, 144
  infection of 106, 173
  transplants 146
  zidovudine and 147, 154
Bowen, Otis 20, 57, 60
brain, infection of 106–7, 120, 144,
  173
Brazil 20, 211–12
breast milk 131, 135, 136–7
Britain
  blood supply 22–3, 68, 87, 88,
    134
  costs of AIDS 21, 22, 23, 155–6
  education 22, 250–51, 259

270